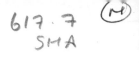

Eye Disease in Clinical Practice

A CONCISE COLOUR ATLAS

Eye Disease in Clinical Practice

A CONCISE COLOUR ATLAS

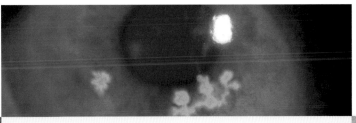

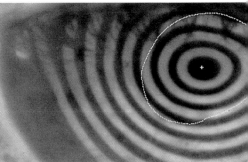

Peter Shah BSc (Hons) MB ChB FRCOphth

Andrew S Jacks OStJ BSc FRCOphth

Peng T Khaw PhD FRCP FRCS FRCOphth

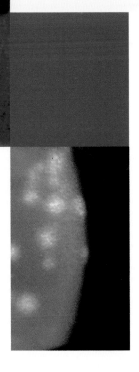

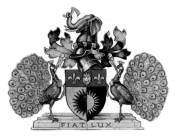

FIAT LUX

PUBLISHED IN ASSOCIATION
WITH MOORFIELDS EYE
HOSPITAL NHS TRUST, LONDON

MANTICORE EUROPE LIMITED

First published in Great Britain in 1999 by Manticore Europe Limited
Silver Birches, Heronsgate, Rickmansworth, Herts. WD3 5DN

British Library Cataloguing in Publication Data
A CIP record for this book is available from the British Library
ISBN 1 900887 03 7

PRINTED AND BOUND IN GREAT BRITAIN BY BATH PRESS LIMITED, GLASGOW

THE MOORFIELDS EYE HOSPITAL COAT OF ARMS

Many of the allusions in the hospital arms need no explanation: the sun
counterchanged, representing darkness giving way to light, the fleam or surgeon's
lancet, the peacocks with their multiple 'eyes', and the ophthalmoscopes. The
leopard's head and the fleur-de-lys are found respectively in the arms of Guy's
Hospital and St Thomas' Hospital in recognition of the staffs of these hospitals
who suggested the founding of the hospital. The elephant's head is in reference
to John Cunningham Saunders the founder of the hospital and appears on many
Saunders arms. The Latin motto reads 'Let there be light'.

*This book is dedicated
to our parents and wives*

Inside the front cover of this book, you will find a CD-ROM. The CD has been published to enable you to view the book on your computer and take advantage of the interactive links, magnification and search facility and other navigational tools.

Important Notice

The terms and conditions of using this CD-ROM are set out on the CD under the heading 'Copyright Notice and Terms and Conditions of Use'.

It is a prerequisite of using this CD-ROM that you read the Terms and Conditions of Use, and by proceeding to access the CD-ROM, you agree to be bound by the terms and conditions as set out in the licence agreement. All terms and conditions are governed by the laws of England.

System Requirements

- PC – 486 or higher with Windows™ 95 or 98
- Mac – Power PC processor with Mac OS 7.6 or higher
- Both platforms require Adobe Acrobat® to read the pages. If you do not have Adobe Acrobat® installed on your computer, the CD contains the software which can be installed free of charge.

Instructions for running the CD

- Insert the CD in the computer
- Double click on the CD-ROM icon to open it (Mac), or click the START button and select RUN from the menu. Type your CD-ROM drive access code and click the OK button (PC)
- If necessary install Adobe Acrobat® using the instructions on the screen
- Read or print out the *Read Me* file for detailed instructions
- Click in the *Eye Disease* icon to open the book

Using the book

There are four choices on the opening page:
1. Copyright Notice and Terms and Conditions of Use
2. About Moorfields Eye Hospital
3. Eye Disease in Clinical Practice
4. Index

The CD displays each page of the book on the right-hand half of the split screen. In this mode, the various chapters of the book are displayed on the left-hand side.

Click on the control triangle to the left of the chapter name and you will open or close the page contents of the chapter; click on any page and you will open the page on the right-hand display. Other, detailed instructions for using the navigational tools are to be found by using the help facility.

Contents

USING THE CD-ROM 6

AUTHOR BIOGRAPHIES 8

FOREWORD 9

ACKNOWLEDGEMENTS 10

1	Introduction 11
2	Embryology 13
3	Anatomy 15
4	Clinical Examination – Tools 19
5	Refractive Errors 33
6	The Eyelids, Orbit and Lacrimal System 37
7	The Conjunctiva, Cornea and Sclera 55
8	Glaucoma 73
9	Uveitis 81
10	The Lens 87
11	Retinal and Macular Disease 93
12	Ocular Oncology 111
13	Strabismus 115
14	Paediatric Ophthalmology 121
15	Neuro-ophthalmology 129
16	Surgical Procedures 143

APPENDIX 1 172

APPENDIX 2 173

INDEX 174

Mr Peter Shah BSc(Hons) MB ChB FRCOphth
Senior Registrar/Fellow in Ophthalmology, Moorfields Eye Hospital, London

Mr Shah has recently been appointed a consultant ophthalmic surgeon to Good Hope Hospital NHS Trust (Birmingham) and the Birmingham & Midland Eye Centre. He is currently a Senior Registrar in Ophthalmology at Moorfields Eye Hospital and is working as a Fellow on the Glaucoma Service. He has previously held posts in general medicine, general surgery, neurosurgery and accident and emergency medicine. Ophthalmology training has been completed in Leeds, Birmingham, Brisbane and London. His sub-specialist area of interest within ophthalmology is adult and developmental glaucoma.

Mr Shah has written approximately 50 papers, chapters and books, and is one of the co-authors of *Key Topics in Ophthalmology* – a postgraduate textbook written for candidates preparing for the final Fellowship of the Royal College of Ophthalmologists. He is actively involved in teaching and has designed and run national courses in ophthalmic education.

Mr Andrew S Jacks OStJ BSc FRCOphth
Specialist Registrar in Ophthalmology, Moorfields Eye Hospital, London

Mr Jacks is a Specialist Registrar in Ophthalmology at Moorfields Eye Hospital. Having graduated from St Thomas' Hospital, London, he took up a commission in the Royal Army Medical Corps. This led to service in South Armagh, Northern Ireland as medical officer to the Coldstream Guards for which he was awarded a General Officer Commanding commendation and also in the former Yugoslavia with the United Nations for which he was awarded the Order of St John for humanitarian services. Mr Jacks' special interests include trauma, strabismus and neuro-ophthalmology and he has recently returned from a one-year secondment in South Africa studying ophthalmic trauma. He was awarded the Harcourt medal for the final fellowship examination.

Mr Jacks has written articles on ophthalmology; he teaches ophthalmologists, nurses, medical students and optometrists and has been a lecturer on several courses.

Professor PT Khaw PhD FRCP FRCS FRCOphth
Professor and Consultant Ophthalmic Surgeon, Glaucoma Unit,
Moorfields Eye Hospital and Wound Healing Research Unit, Dept. of Pathology,
Institute of Ophthalmology, London

Professor Khaw is Professor and Consultant Ophthalmic Surgeon at Moorfields Eye Hospital. Before specialising in ophthalmology, he trained in general medicine and was formerly Lecturer in Ophthalmology at Southampton University before becoming Senior Registrar and then Consultant at Moorfields Eye Hospital. He was also a Wellcome Trust Research Fellow during which time he carried out a PhD in cellular and molecular biology of ocular wound healing.

Professor Khaw has been involved in teaching medical students and general practitioners, ophthalmologists, optometrists and nurses throughout his career. He has published over 200 papers, chapters and books including the *ABC of Eyes*, which is currently the best selling general ophthalmology book in the United Kingdom.

It is a pleasure to introduce *Eye Disease in Clinical Practice: a Concise Colour Atlas*, not only because it lives up to its title by being concise and very colourful, but most of all because it fills an important gap in the literary armamentarium of the general physician. Exposure to ophthalmology during undergraduate medical training is sparse – certainly insufficient to carry the clinician through the many years of practice which lie ahead. More the pity because eye problems are very common in general practice and many have systemic implications.

This colour atlas is ideal to acquaint or refresh the busy clinician on a vast range of ophthalmic conditions, and also on up-to-date methods of examination and state of the art treatments. This will be helpful during discussions with patients, some of whom will be armed with the latest colour supplement or information from the web.

The picture-based approach with short accompanying texts makes the book particularly accessible and easy to dip into. With over 200 stunning illustrations and flow charts, all the major topics and more are covered. Subjects are sensibly weighted for everyday practice and those eye conditions with systemic associations and implications receive special emphasis.

Eye Disease in Clinical Practice: a Concise Colour Atlas by Peter Shah, Andrew Jacks and Peng Khaw is superb, and offers a new insight into the fascinating subject of ophthalmology, with its unique blend of medicine and surgery. This is not a book to look after or worse still to lock away in a remote library cabinet. Use it, keep it close at hand, so that it is there when you or your colleagues most need it – when the patient presents.

Alistair R Fielder
FRCP FRCS FRCOphth
Professor of Ophthalmology
Imperial College School of Medicine
London

Acknowledgements

Designing and writing an atlas is a huge undertaking and it is not possible without the help of many people. We should like to extend special thanks to: Mr Alan Lacey for his superb technical artistic work; Miss Gill Adams for helping to organise several illustrations which were difficult to obtain; Professor Alistair Fielder for his invaluable comments, ideas and kind foreword; and finally to Mr Richard Warman for his tremendous patience, meticulous attention to detail and good humour.

We are also grateful to the following people for their help during the preparation of this atlas:

I. Balmer	P. Hamilton	J. Morin	G. Smith
G. Banerjee	G. Holder	R. Poynter	J. Stevens
M. Collins	P. Khaw	A. Rauf	A. Sullivan
M. Connor	L. Lane	M. Restori	T. Watts
C. Contrino	R. Leung	N. Sapp	M. Wearne
C. Daniel	C. Martin	K. Sehmi	
D. Gartry	A. McIntyre	A. Singh	

PS, ASJ, PTK

1 Introduction

Eye Disease in Clinical Practice: A Concise Colour Atlas comprehensively covers the more common and important ophthalmic conditions a clinician will encounter in their practice. Many health care professionals commonly see patients with eye disease. The examination of these patients and making a diagnosis can be a great challenge. For example, the 'Top 50' differential diagnoses for the red eye are listed in Appendix 2.

The aim of this book is to make ophthalmology a more friendly subject to medical and paramedical clinicians, and hopefully their patients. The main feature on each page is a high quality colour image of the topic under discussion. Where relevant, the image is accompanied by a life-size image of the condition. This has been done so that the reader can appreciate some of the difficulties involved with the diagnosis in situations where they may not have access to sophisticated ophthalmic equipment.

Each image is accompanied by concise text, describing the conditions and physical signs present. Important information about the disease, including the urgency of referral, is highlighted. Each condition is referenced in the index and the common abbreviations are listed in Appendix 1 at page 172. Common techniques of ophthalmic examination and investigation together with a range of modern ophthalmic operations are also covered, enabling discussion of the procedures that the patient may undergo. This allows the book to be used as a working tool to aid patient consultation, helping the patient to prepare for their ophthalmic examination or operation, using the high-resolution colour images.

This book is aimed at all health care professionals who deal with ophthalmic problems, including: Ophthalmologists, General Practitioners, Optometrists, Ophthalmic Nurses, Ophthalmic Secretaries, Undergraduate Medical Students, Post-graduate Clinicians in related specialities (General Medicine, Neurology) and Clinicians in Accident & Emergency Departments.

2.1 Embryology of the Eye

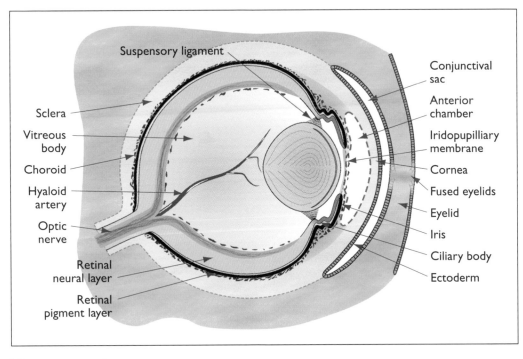

Suspensory ligament

Sclera

Vitreous body

Choroid

Hyaloid artery

Optic nerve

Retinal neural layer

Retinal pigment layer

Conjunctival sac

Anterior chamber

Iridopupilliary membrane

Cornea

Fused eyelids

Eyelid

Iris

Ciliary body

Ectoderm

The eye at 15 weeks

The antero-posterior (A–P) section above shows the eye at the 15-week stage of development. Most of the key elements in the eye are already at an advanced stage of development when the embryo is only 15 weeks old (into the start of the second trimester). **Intrauterine infection**, for example, rubella, **maternal drug ingestion**, and **alcohol** abuse may have serious effects on the eye at this time. It is important to look for developmental anomalies of the eye in the post-natal examination. The anterior segment continues to alter until the age of about 4 years, and the posterior segment may continue growing until the age of about 16 years. There is a wide spectrum of developmental anomalies some of which are shown overleaf together with a table of embryological development.

2.2 Embryology – Key Dates

Developmental Anomalies

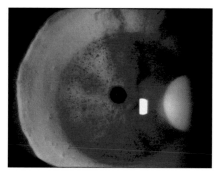

Congenital cataract present in central area of lens (nucleus) (see 14.3)

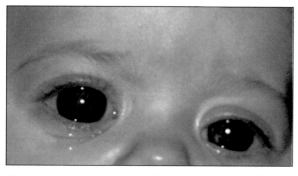

Congenital glaucoma – raised intraocular pressure due to failure of development of drainage channels. (see 14.6)

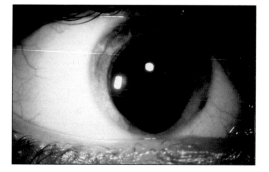

Iris coloboma – due to failure of complete closure of inferior fissure in eye

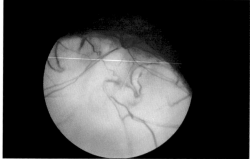

Posterior segment coloboma – due to failure of inferior half of eye to fuse

Duration of Gestation	Development of the Eye	Related Congenital Defect
22 days	*Formation of optic vesicles from forebrain; invagination of cleft for hyaloid artery*	Anophthalmia/coloboma
23 days	*Retina starts to form*	Retinal agenesis or malformation
27 days	*Lens and retinal vessels start to form*	Cataract
32 days	*Cornea starts to form*	Corneal scarring
35 days	*Invagination of lacrimal system begins*	Periorbital cleft/fistula or system not patent
45 days	*Trabecular meshwork starts to form*	Glaucoma
20–22 weeks	*Upper and lower lids begin to separate*	Ankyloblepharon (fused eyelids)
30 weeks	*Regression of hyaloid artery commences*	Persistent hyaloid artery
34–36 weeks	*Pupillary membrane regresses*	Persistent pupillary membrane

Table of embryological development

3.1 Parts of the Eye Normally Visible on External Inspection

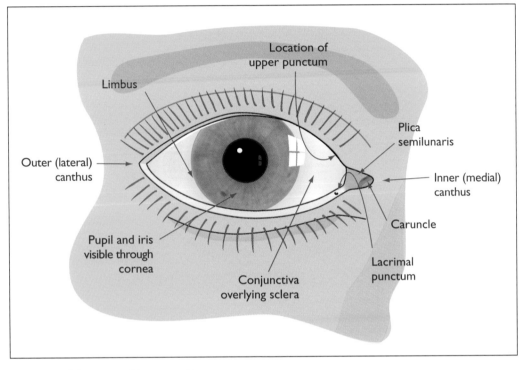

Anatomy of the eye visible externally

When describing the external appearance of the eye, it is important to use the correct anatomical terms to avoid confusion. The central transparent **cornea** with a diameter of approximately 11.5 mm is surrounded by the white **sclera**. The sclera is surrounded by a fibrous (Tenon's) capsule, and the visible anterior portion is covered with **conjunctiva**, a vascular mucous membrane. The central black aperture in the coloured iris is the pupil. The lacrimal drainage system is situated in the medial canthal region. There is a single lacrimal punctum on both the upper and lower lids situated about 5 mm to 6 mm from the medial canthal angle.

3.2 Cross-section through the Eye

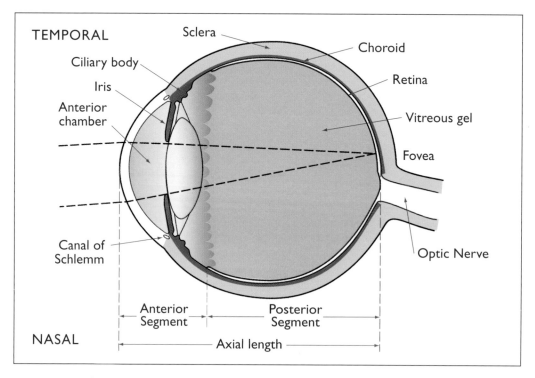

Cross-section of the right eye viewed from above

The eyeball is divided into two main regions: the **anterior segment** comprising the cornea, sclera, anterior chamber, iris, lens and ciliary body; and the **posterior segment** comprising the vitreous gel, retina, choroid, optic nerve head and posterior sclera. The thickness of the posterior adult sclera is 1 mm, but may be as thin as 0.3 mm in places. In normal eyes the **axial length** (distance from the front of the cornea to the retina) is about 22 to 24 mm.

3.3 Posterior Pole – Optic Nerve and Macula

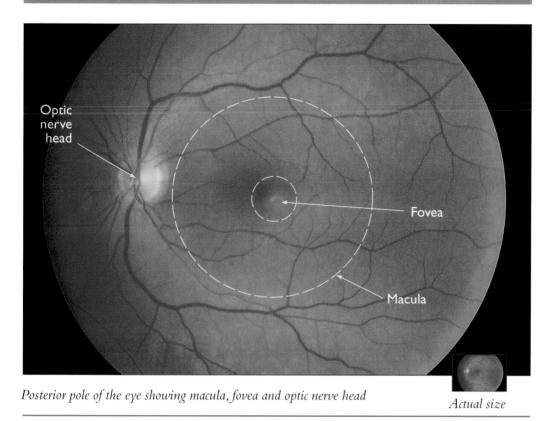

Optic nerve head

Fovea

Macula

Actual size

Posterior pole of the eye showing macula, fovea and optic nerve head

The **macula** is an oval area in the central region of the posterior pole which measures about 4 to 5 mm in diameter. There is a small depression in the centre of the macula measuring 1.5 mm in diameter – the **fovea**. The fovea is the area of retina with greatest sensitivity and resolving power, and consists almost entirely of **cones**, with a photoreceptor density of about 150,000 to 200,000 cones per square millimetre. The **optic nerve head** is approximately 3 mm nasal to the fovea, and measures about 1.5 mm in diameter. There are 1,200,000 axons leaving the eye along the optic nerve.

3.4 Visual Pathway

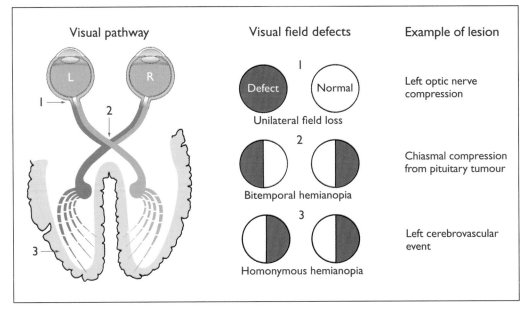

Visual pathway	Visual field defects	Example of lesion

Unilateral field loss — Left optic nerve compression

Bitemporal hemianopia — Chiasmal compression from pituitary tumour

Homonymous hemianopia — Left cerebrovascular event

The visual pathway showing visual field defects resulting from lesions in different locations

The **visual pathway** is the neural connection between the retina and the occipital cortex. The axons from the **retinal ganglion cells** travel along the optic nerve and then **decussate** at the **optic chiasm** and pass to the **lateral geniculate nucleus** (LGN) via the **optic tract**. Fibres then pass along the **optic radiations** from the LGN to the **visual (occipital) cortex**. The decussation at the chiasm means that the left visual hemifield is represented in the right occipital lobe, and the right hemifield in the left occipital lobe. Lesions of the visual pathway produce specific visual field defects depending on the site of the lesion. The figure above shows the effect of lesions at three different sites.

4.1 Vision Testing Chart

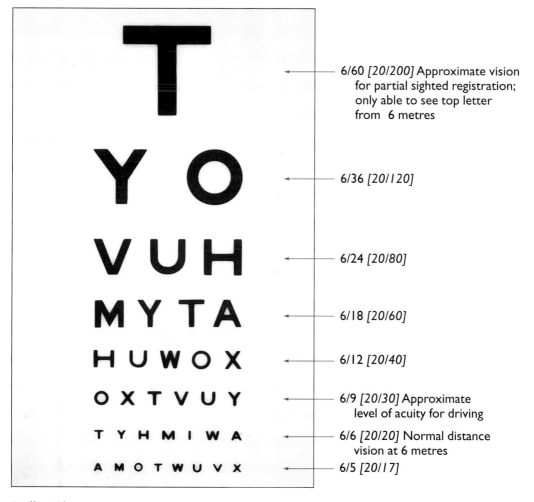

6/60 [20/200] Approximate vision for partial sighted registration; only able to see top letter from 6 metres

6/36 [20/120]

6/24 [20/80]

6/18 [20/60]

6/12 [20/40]

6/9 [20/30] Approximate level of acuity for driving

6/6 [20/20] Normal distance vision at 6 metres

6/5 [20/17]

Snellen Chart

The Snellen Chart is the standard method for measuring **visual acuity** in the United Kingdom. The patient stands **6 metres** from the chart and each eye is tested separately. **Distance glasses** should be worn, but if these are not available a **pin-hole** should be used to estimate the corrected visual acuity. Visual function is expressed as a fraction: the upper (numerator) is the distance in metres from the chart and the lower (denominator) is the number of the lowest line the patient can read. **Normal vision is 6/6**. The notation used in some other countries is shown in square brackets. If visual function is very poor, it can be recorded as the ability to count fingers (CF) or perceive hand movements (HM) or light (PL).

4.2 Infant Vision Testing

Visual Function in Infancy

Age	Testing Visual Function	Approximate Visual Acuity
Newborn	*Fixes and turns towards light* *Pupils respond to light* *Blink response to stimulus* *Visual-evoked potential (see 4.13)*	6/240 [20/800]
1–2 months	*Stable ocular alignment* *Looks and smiles at mother/faces* *Fixes and follows face or toy*	6/180 – 6/90 [20/600 – 20/300]
3–6 months	*Visually directed reaching (unreliable)* *Ability to locate small objects* *(hundreds and thousands)* *Rolling and mounted balls* *(Worth and Stycar)* *Preferential looking (acuity cards)*	6/18 – 6/6 [20/60 – 20/20]
1 year	*Acuity cards* *Matching pictures and optotypes*	6/9 – 6/6 [20/30 – 20/20]
2 years	*Acuity cards* *Matching pictures and optotypes* *Able to name objects*	6/6 [20/20]

Although difficult, it is possible to obtain an **estimate** of visual function in a **pre-verbal** child. Much useful information about vision can be gained by talking to the **parents** and simply **observing** the child. If visual function is equal in both eyes, then the child will not object to either eye being **occluded**.

4.3 Infant Vision Testing

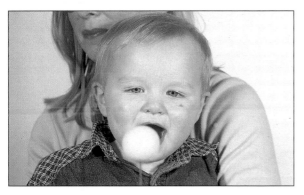

6 month old child fixing and following a Stycar ball

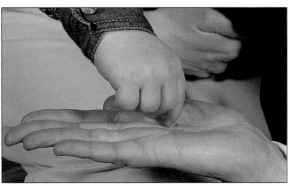

6 month old child picking up a hundreds and thousands sweet

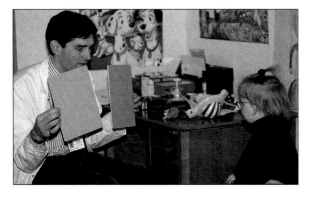

2 year old child being tested with Cardiff acuity cards

Visual development is a complex maturation process, which continues throughout infancy. Whilst it is desirable to **quantify** visual acuity in a standard Snellen notation, visual function in infants is often assessed with qualitative tests. **Measurement** of vision in children of less than one year is possible using the techniques of **forced choice preferential looking** and the **visually evoked response**. Testing vision in infants is difficult and time consuming and several attempts are needed to gain reliable assessments.

4.4 Slit-lamp plus 78 Dioptre Lens

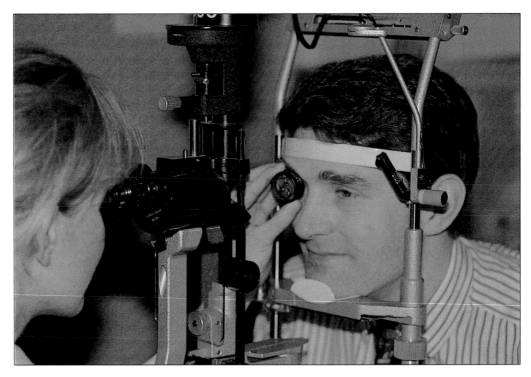

Examination of retina through a 78 dioptre lens using the slit lamp microscope

The slit–lamp (a binocular microscope with variable slit illumination) can be used to examine the anterior segment of the eye in detail and to measure intraocular pressure. In combination with a 78 dioptre (D) lens the slit–lamp can provide a highly magnified view of the retina. It is often necessary to **dilate the pupils**, for example, with G.Tropicamide 1% (eye drops), to examine the retina in detail, and this results in **blurring** of the patient's vision for up to 6 hours until the effect wears off. Therefore, patients are usually advised not to drive until normal vision returns.

4.5 Applanation Tonometry

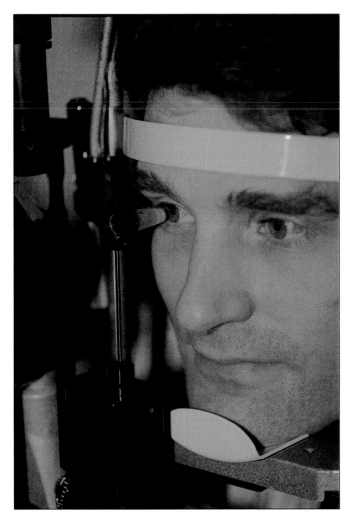

Intraocular pressure being measured using contact applanation tonometry

In the out-patient setting the most accurate way of measuring intraocular pressure (IOP) is to perform **applanation tonometry** at the slit-lamp microscope. After the instillation of a drop of local anaesthetic and fluorescein, the tonometer head is positioned so that it is in contact with a specific area of the cornea. The procedure is rapid and painless.

4.6 Pneumotonometry

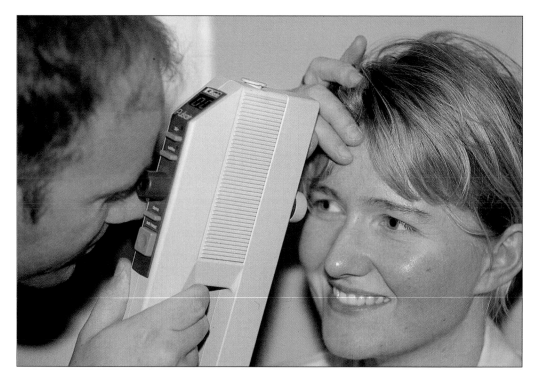

Measurement of intraocular pressure using a pneumotonometer

Pneumotonometry ('air puff') is an alternative technique of measuring intraocular pressure (IOP), which is in common use in many **optometric** practices. During the measurement a small jet of air is directed at the cornea – a procedure which some patients find unpleasant. The main problem with pneumotonometry is that there is a **tendency to overestimate the IOP**, with the result that many patients have an erroneous diagnosis of elevated IOP.

4.7 Direct Ophthalmoscopy

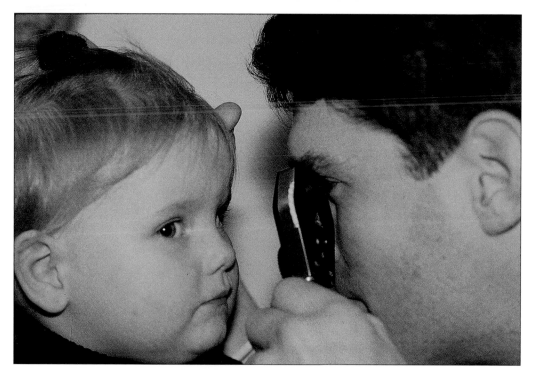

Examination of the fundus using a direct ophthalmoscope

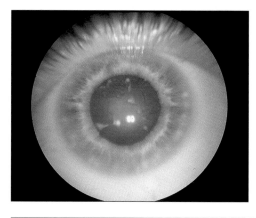

*Red reflex as seen with
a direct ophthalmoscope*

Direct ophthalmoscopy can be performed through an undilated pupil and one can obtain a good view of the optic disc, macula and posterior pole in most patients. The patient should be asked to look into the distance with the other eye. From a distance of about 50 cm, it is also possible to assess the **red reflex**.

4.8 Indirect Ophthalmoscopy

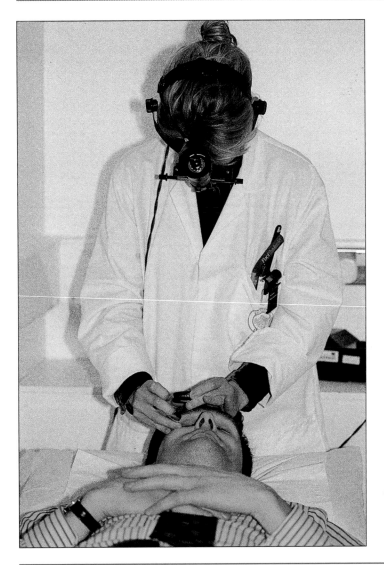

The retina being examined with a head mounted indirect ophthalmoscope

In order to perform a detailed examination of the retina, for example, in a case of possible retinal detachment, it is necessary to have a maximally dilated pupil and to use the technique of **indirect ophthalmoscopy**. A 20 or 28 dioptre lens is used in combination with a head-mounted light source and optical system. In order to visualise the most peripheral, anterior regions of the retina it is often necessary to **indent** the eye under local anaesthesia with a scleral indentor.

4.9 Assessment of the Red Reflex

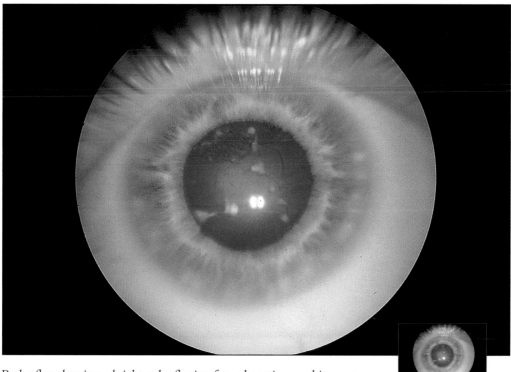

Red reflex showing a bright red reflection from the retina – white spots indicate mild cataract

Actual size

Assessment of the **red reflex** through a dilated pupil can provide useful information about the presence of ocular pathology. The red reflex is viewed as light reflecting back from a pink healthy retina with a **direct ophthalmoscope** from a distance of about 50 cm (see 4.7). If the red reflex is obscured, it may indicate the presence of dense **cataract** or **vitreous haemorrhage**. Posterior subcapsular cataract may appear as a black opacity in the centre of the red reflex. Similarly, one may see the radiating 'spoke-like' black opacities of cortical cataract in the reflex. If the reflex appears **white** (leukocoria - see 14.2) instead of red, this may indicate posterior segment pathology such as retinoblastoma or retino–choroidal coloboma.

4.10 Testing Visual Fields to Confrontation

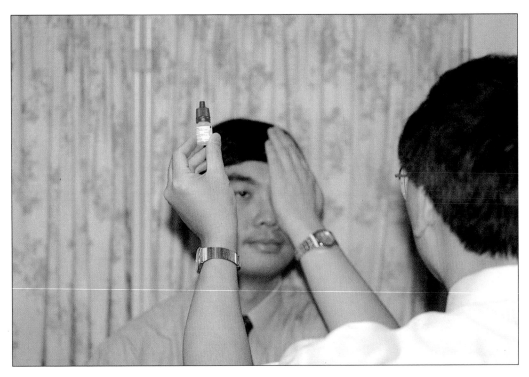

Visual field being tested using red target

Testing visual fields to confrontation can be performed very rapidly and can be extremely helpful in assessing patients who present with visual loss. The examiner should be seated about **one metre** from the patient and their face should be at the same level. Testing each eye separately, the examiner **compares** the visual field of the patient with his own, by bringing a target, for example, a **5 mm red pin**, from the **peripheral field towards fixation** in each **quadrant** of vision.

4.11 Automated Visual Field Testing

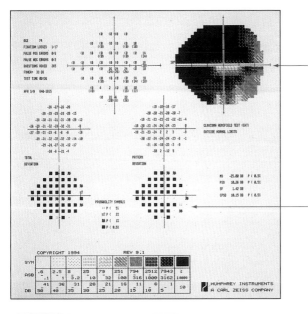

Greyscale analysis of retinal sensitivity to light in central 30° field:

Black = areas of total field loss

Grey = areas of partial field loss

White = areas of normal visual field

Plot to show the statistical significance of areas of field loss:

Black square = statistically significant

The printout shown (advanced glaucoma) enables rapid analysis of a visual field defect. The two areas indicated above on the printout are the key indicators of damage

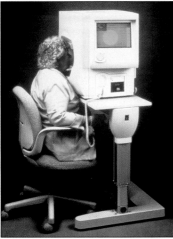

Patient undergoing visual field testing on a computerised perimeter

Automated visual field testing provides an accurate, repeatable and quantifiable assessment of the **central visual field**. This method of analysis is particularly useful in monitoring patients with **glaucoma** (see 8.6) and **neurological disease** (see 15.4 and 15.5). The technique is only suitable for patients who are able to co-operate and perform the test reliably; some elderly patients have difficulty maintaining concentration for the full test duration. Computerised perimetry is now the standard method of sequentially testing visual fields in ophthalmic practice.

4.12 Ultrasonography

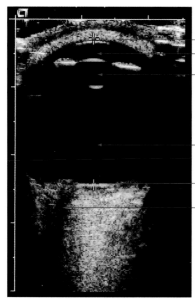

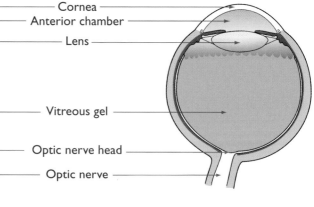

Cornea
Anterior chamber
Lens

Vitreous gel

Optic nerve head

Optic nerve

Ultrasound of the normal eye

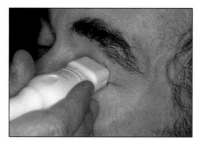

Ultrasound probe resting gently on closed eyelids

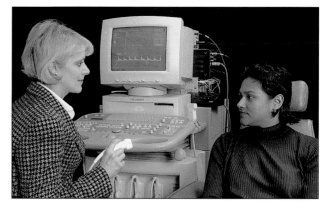

Ultrasonic equipment

Ocular ultrasonography is used for two main purposes. First, to visualise the posterior segment of the eye, for example, to exclude a retinal detachment, or when media opacity such as cataract or vitreous haemorrhage impair the direct view. Secondly, to make accurate measurements of the axial length of the eye, when calculating the power of the intraocular lens needed for cataract surgery. Ultrasonography is a quick and painless procedure.

4.13 Electrodiagnostic Testing

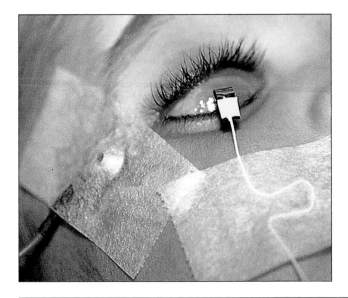

Child with opaque corneas undergoing electrodiagnostic testing under anaesthetic to test retinal function

Electrodiagnostic tests provide an objective means of assessing the **function** of the visual pathway. The **visual-evoked potential** (VEP) can be used to assess optic nerve function, for example, in demyelination, and can help to differentiate between organic and functional causes of visual loss, for example, in cases of malingering. **Electroretinography** (ERG) and **electro-oculography** (EOG) are techniques that provide information about the function of the various component layers of the retina. The EOG and ERG may aid diagnosis in cases of retinal or macular dystrophy.

Electrodiagnostic Testing Chart

Type of Test	The Test	Uses of the Test
Visually Evoked Response (VER or VEP)	*The electrical potential generated by the occipital (visual) cortex in response to stimulation of the retina by light*	Diagnosis of optic nerve disease (e.g. demyelination) Evaluation of macular disease Assessment of visual acuity in young children Assessment of visual potential in eyes with opaque media Objective aid in diagnosing malingering patients
Electroretinogram (ERG)	*The electrical potential generated by the retinal stimulation of the retina by light*	Assessment of retinal function in eyes with opaque media *photoreceptors and bipolar cells in response to* (e.g. dense cataract) Assessment of infants who are functionally blind, with no visible retinal pathology (e.g. Leber's amaurosis) Assessment of retinal dystrophies (e.g. retinitis pigmentosa) Assessment of night blindness Investigation of maculopathies
Electro-oculogram (EOG)	*The resting electrical potential between the front (cornea) and back of the eye, generated by the retinal pigment epithelium and photoreceptors*	Investigation of maculopathies (e.g. Stargardt's disease) Assessment of 'carriers' in inherited maculopathies Assessment of retinal dystrophies Assessment of night blindness

Electrodiagnostic testing chart

4.14 Fundus Fluorescein Angiography

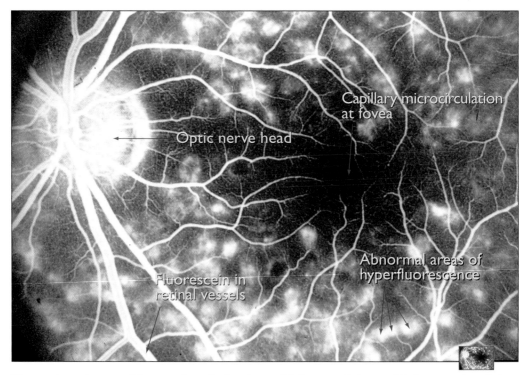

Optic nerve head

Capillary microcirculation at fovea

Abnormal areas of hyperfluorescence

Fluorescein in retinal vessels

Fluorescein angiogram of the posterior pole showing multiple areas of abnormal leakage   *Actual size*

Fundus fluorescein angiography (FFA) is a diagnostic technique used to provide information about diseases of the posterior segment of the eye. The patient is seated at a fundus camera and given an **intravenous** injection of fluorescein, after which a rapid sequence of photographs are taken as fluorescein enters the **choroidal** and **retinal circulations**. The dye fluoresces under conditions of excitation with blue light, and the state of the **blood-ocular barrier** can be accurately assessed. FFA can identify abnormal blood vessels, abnormal areas of dye leakage and areas of retinal ischaemia. FFA results in a temporary change in the colour of the patient's skin, urine and tears. This may stain soft contact lenses.

5 Refractive Errors

5.1 Myopia

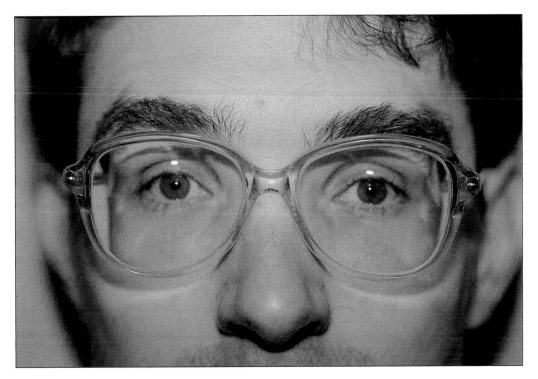

Myopic glasses – the face and eyes appear smaller behind the lenses

Patients who are **myopic** (short-sighted) tend to have an eye with an axial length that is **longer** than normal. Light from distant objects is focused in front of the retina, which produces a blurred image. Myopes usually have reasonable unaided near vision. Optical correction with glasses or contact lenses requires a **concave ('minus')** lens. When someone wears a myopic spectacle correction their eyes and face appear **reduced in size** to an observer looking at them. Patients with moderate and high myopia have an increased risk of developing a **retinal detachment** (see 11.1) and **open angle glaucoma** (see 8.2). Progressive pathological myopia is also associated with macular disease and is a significant cause of blind registration.

5.2 Hypermetropia

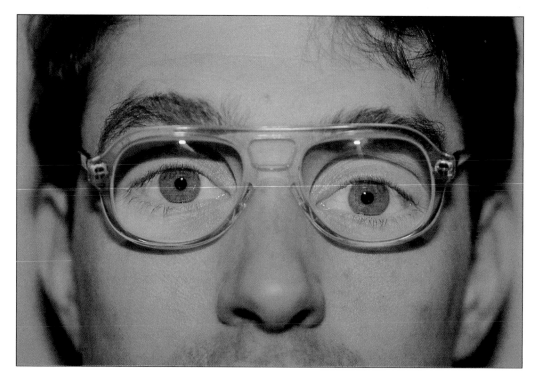

Hypermetropic glasses – the face and eyes appear larger behind the lenses

Patients who are **hypermetropic** (long-sighted) tend to have an eye with an axial length that is **shorter** than normal. Light from distant objects is focused behind the retina, but by changing the shape of the crystalline lens, known as accommodation, younger patients can bring the image into focus. As the power of accommodation declines with advancing age (see 5.3), the hypermetrope finds it increasingly difficult to focus and requires a **convex ('plus')** lens for optical correction. When someone wears a hypermetropic spectacle correction their eyes and face appear **magnified** to an observer looking at them. Patients with moderate and high hypermetropia have an increased risk of developing both **acute and chronic angle-closure glaucoma** (see 8.1 and 8.2).

5 Refractive Errors

5.3 Presbyopia

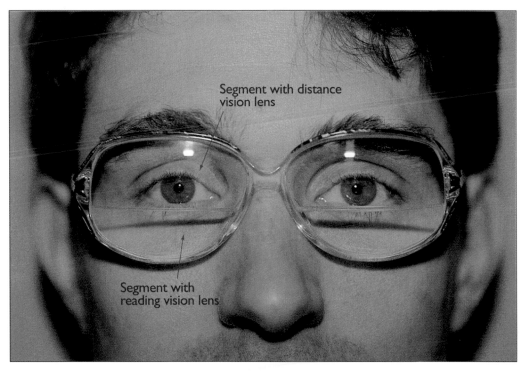

Segment with distance vision lens

Segment with reading vision lens

Bifocal glasses — inferior half of lens corrects presbyopia

When someone with a normal (emmetropic) eye needs to focus on a near object, the shape of the crystalline lens is altered to make it more convex and increasing its refractive power. The ability to **accommodate** starts to significantly **decline in middle-age**. This is known as **presbyopia** and patients notice that they find it **increasingly difficult to read**. Patients with early presbyopia notice that they need to hold books and newspapers further away from their face in order to read clearly. The use of reading glasses with a **convex ('plus')** lens can compensate for the reduction in accommodation. Alternatively, the subject may have bifocal lenses fitted to their glasses.

5.4 Astigmatism

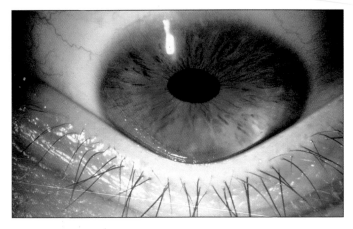

Eye with keratoconus showing cone shaped cornea indenting lower lid

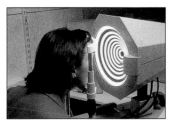

Reflected image of rings on cornea show oval shape which indicates astigmatism

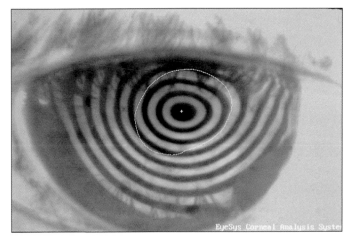

Measuring corneal astigmatism

In a normal eye the **cornea** is the major refractive element involved in producing a focused image. The surface of the cornea should approximate to part of a **sphere** producing a clear retinal image. When an eye has an **astigmatic error** the surface of the cornea is not spherical, but rather part of a **rugby shaped ball** where **one meridian has a greater refractive power than the other**, thereby resulting in the production of a blurred retinal image. Astigmatism may occur in combination with another refractive error, for example, with myopia; in association with corneal disease, for example, with keratoconus – shown above; or following ocular **surgery**, for example, for cataract. Special **cylindrical** lenses can be incorporated into glasses to correct astigmatism.

6.1 Basal Cell Carcinoma

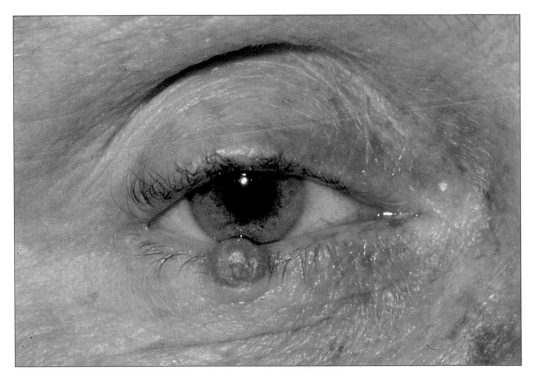

Lower lid basal cell carcinoma seen as ulcerated raised lesion

Basal cell carcinomas ('rodent ulcers') are the most common periorbital neoplasm and 70% occur in the region of the **lower eyelid**. The most important risk factor is **actinic** damage in fair-skinned individuals. Lesions are usually painless and present as nodular or plaque-like areas with irregular, rolled 'pearly' edges, with associated telangectasia and central ulceration. Metastasis is **rare**. The principle of management is to achieve **complete excision**, to avoid destructive **local invasion** of the orbit and central nervous system. **Histopathological diagnosis is essential**.

6.2 Squamous Cell Carcinoma

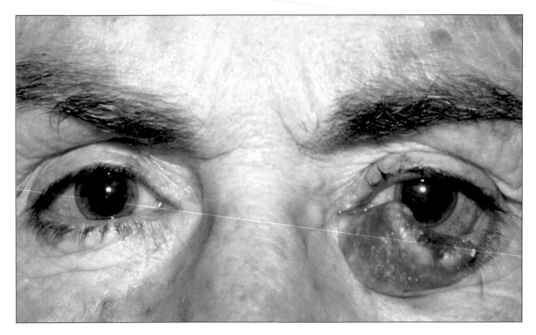

Squamous cell carcinoma invading left lower lid

Most **squamous cell carcinomas** (sccs) arise from pre-existing lesions such as an area of **actinic keratosis**. Lesions may appear very similar to those seen in basal cell carcinoma, often with more scaling and fissuring of the skin. The key to the management of sccs is to make an **early diagnosis**, because of the potential for **metastasis**. It is essential to achieve complete excision of the lesion, and this often means that an extensive oculoplastic lid reconstruction is required. **Histopathological diagnosis is essential**.

6.3 Entropion

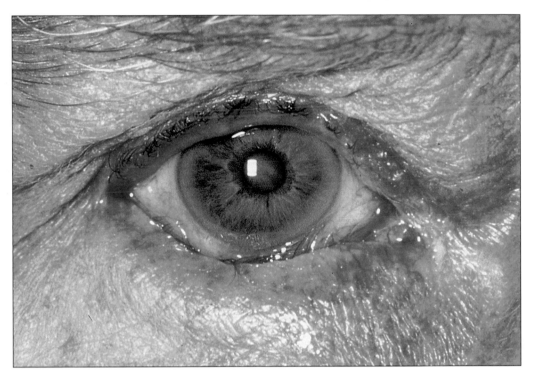

Lower lid entropion with in-turned lashes rubbing on eye

Entropion is a **malposition** of the eyelid (usually lower) in which the lid margin is **turned inwards** towards the globe, and the lashes abrade the cornea. Entropion may be **intermittent** and only demonstrable on forcible lid closure. The most common cause of entropion is **aging** (involutional) change of the lid tissues, but scarring (cicatricial) processes can also alter the position of the lid margin. The definitive management of entropion is **surgical correction** (see 16.19).

6.4 Ectropion

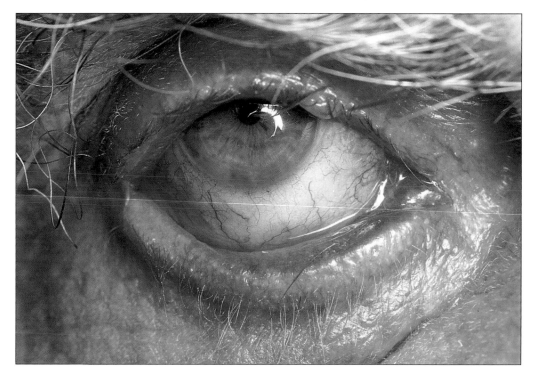

Lower lid ectropion with lower eyelid rotated away from eye

Ectropion is an eyelid **malposition** in which the lid margin is rotated away from the globe and is no longer in correct apposition with the ocular surface. **Aging** (involutional) changes of the lid tissues, **cicatricial** processes and **paralysis** of the **seventh cranial nerve** (see 15.9) are common causes of ectropion. Ectropion may lead to lagophthalmos and **corneal exposure**, hypertrophy of the conjunctiva and **epiphora**. The definitive management is **surgical correction** (see 16.18).

6.5 Ptosis

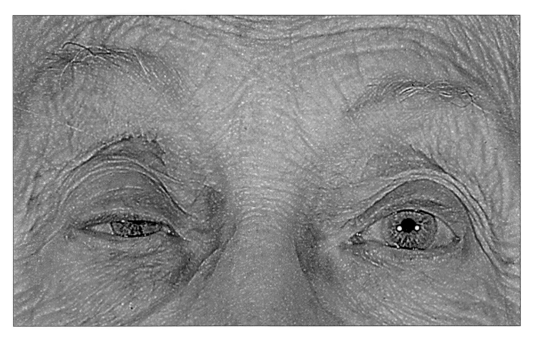

Senile ptosis – drooping of right upper eyelid and wrinkling of forehead

The term **ptosis** is used to describe **malposition** of the upper eyelid in which the lid position is abnormally **low**. Ptosis may be **congenital** (see 14.8) or **acquired**. Acquired causes include **senile** (involutional) changes in the levator muscle/aponeurosis; **myogenic** diseases, for example, myasthenia gravis (see 15.13); **neurogenic** pathology, for example, third cranial nerve palsy (see 15.6) and Horner's syndrome (see 15.12); and traumatic and mechanical causes. **Senile** ptosis, shown above, is associated with a high upper lid crease and frontalis overaction with raised eyebrows.

6.6   Trichiasis

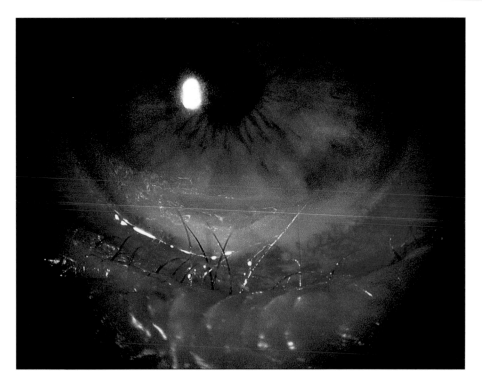

In-turning lashes abrading cornea causing scaring

In trichiasis lashes are turned **inwards** against the globe which causes an uncomfortable, chronic gritty sensation. Persistent **trichiasis** leads to **corneal epithelial damage** (identified by staining with minims fluorescein) and scarring. Causes of trichiasis include **cicatricial** lid diseases such as trauma, trachoma, pemphigoid and rosacea. Management options include **recurrent epilation** (manual removal with forceps), **electrolysis** (electrical destruction of follicles) and lid **cryotherapy** (freezing).

6.7 Allergic Dermatitis

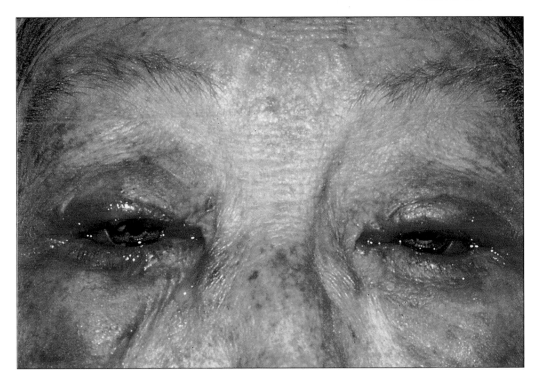

Bilateral allergic dermatitis caused by eye drops

Allergic dermatitis is seen most commonly in association with an allergic reaction to a component of an **eye drop**, either the **active drug** or one of the **preservative** compounds. The periocular skin has an **eczematous**-type reaction with erythema, oedema, scaling and fissuring of the lid skin, and marked **itching**. The most effective treatment is to **stop** all topical drops and use a simple **emollient** on the skin. It takes several weeks for full recovery.

6.8 Blepharitis

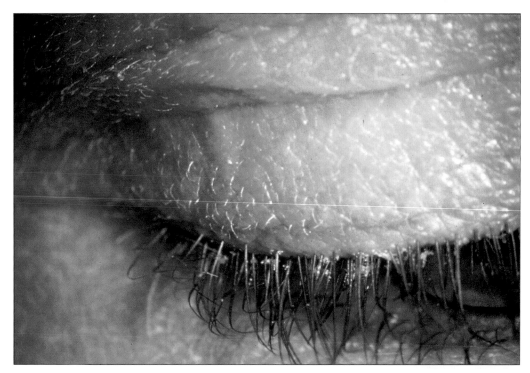

Blepharitis – desquamation around eyelashes

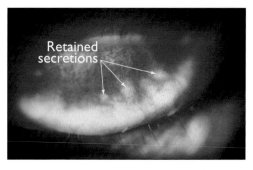
Retained secretions

Retention of secretion within Meibomian glands

Blepharitis is an extremely common **chronic inflammatory** condition affecting the **eyelid margins**. Patients complain of sore, gritty eyes. Lid margin disease may be anterior, with crusting and desquamation around lash follicles or posterior with retention of secretion, plugging the Meibomian glands. Blepharitis is also associated with certain dermatological conditions including **rosacea** and **atopic dermatitis**. Treatment includes: **regular lid hygiene**, **systemic tetracycline**, topical antibiotics and steroids.

6.9 Meibomian Cyst

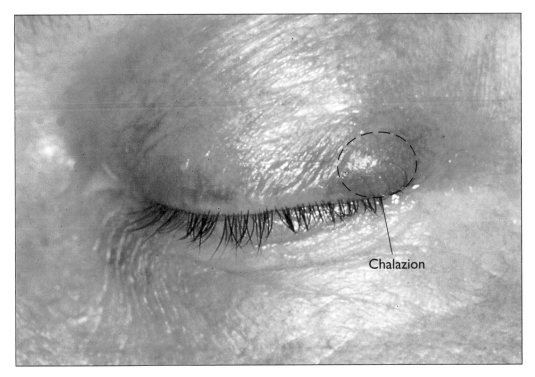

Chalazion

Upper lid chalazion – blocked and inflamed Meibomian gland

Within the tarsal plates of the upper and lower lids there are a series of **Meibomian glands** which secrete lipids involved in stabilising the tear film. These glands can become blocked, particularly if **blepharitis** (see 6.8) is present. Patients usually present with acute onset of a red, painful, swollen lid; and the inflamed 'pea-sized' cystic area (chalazion) is often apparent. If initial treatment with **hot compresses** and **antibiotics** is not successful, ophthalmic referral is needed for cyst incision and curettage (see 16.21).

6.10 Preseptal Cellulitis

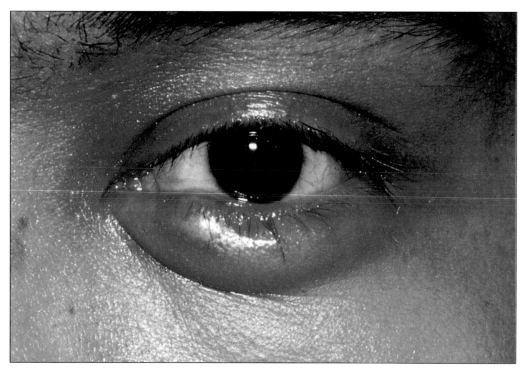

Lid swollen but eye and eye movements normal

Preseptal cellulitis is an **infection** of the tissues **anterior to the orbital septum**. The orbital contents are not involved in the process in contrast to orbital cellulitis (see 6.11). There is often a history of periorbital trauma or signs of a **focus** of infection, for example, a lid margin sty. It is extremely important to **exclude** signs of orbital cellulitis. **Systemic antibiotics** are the treatment of choice.

6.11 Orbital Cellulitis

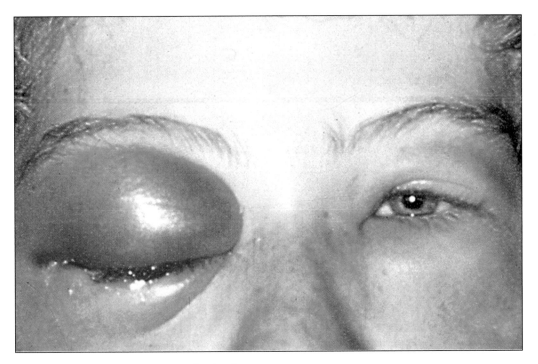

Swollen lid hides life threatening orbital infection

Orbital cellulitis, the infection of the orbital contents posterior to the orbital septum, is an emergency condition. Patients often have marked pain, pyrexia, proptosis, reduced vision, restriction of extraocular movements and lid swelling. There may be an associated infection of the paranasal sinuses which may need surgical drainage. Urgent (same day) admission for investigation of the underlying cause and medical management is required. If left untreated, the following outcomes are possible: a) a 40% mortality rate due to intracranial infection and cavernous sinus thrombosis, and b) blindness.

6.12 Herpes Zoster Ophthalmicus

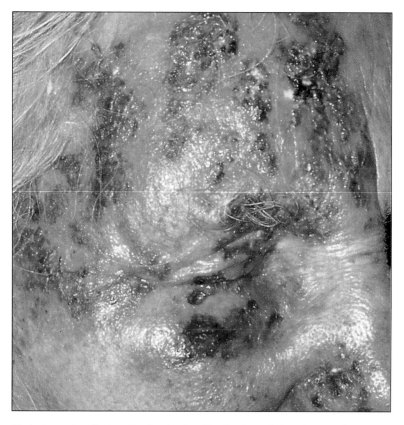

Vesicular rash affecting the face in the distribution of the trigeminal nerve

Herpes zoster ophthalmicus (HZO) is a severe infection of the tissues of the eye, orbit, periorbital region and skin in the distribution of the first division of the trigeminal nerve due to the Herpes zoster virus. Features include a severe eruptive vesicular rash with **conjunctivitis**, **keratitis** and **anterior uveitis**. Ocular disease may result in permanent reduction of visual function; if the skin of the nose is affected, this indicates a higher chance of ocular involvement. If HZO is suspected in the early stages of the disease, **systemic antiviral therapy** may be very helpful in limiting disease duration and **post-herpetic neuralgia**

6.13 Thyroid Eye Disease – Clinical

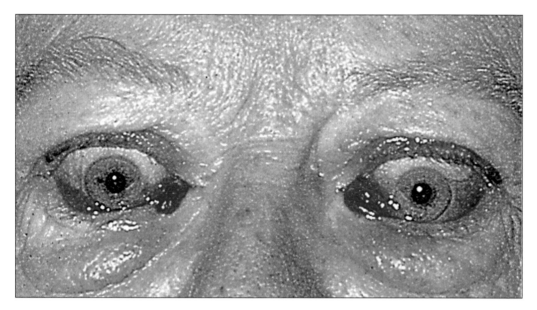

Bilateral thyroid eye disease with exophthalmos and conjunctival oedema (chemosis)

Hyperthyroidism is associated with both lid retraction and lid lag. **Thyroid eye disease** (TED) is an autoimmune condition in which there is an inflammatory lymphocytic infiltration of orbital tissues, especially **orbital fat** and **extraocular muscles**, with increased fibroblast activity and glycosaminoglycan deposition. TED may lead to swelling of the lids, proptosis, restriction of extraocular movements and optic nerve compression (see 6.14). Thyroid eye disease is the most common cause of both unilateral and bilateral **proptosis**. Patients with TED may be hypothyroid, euthyroid or hyperthyroid. TED may follow treatment of hyperthyroidism with radioactive iodine (I^{131}).

6.14 Thyroid Eye Disease – Radiology of the Orbit

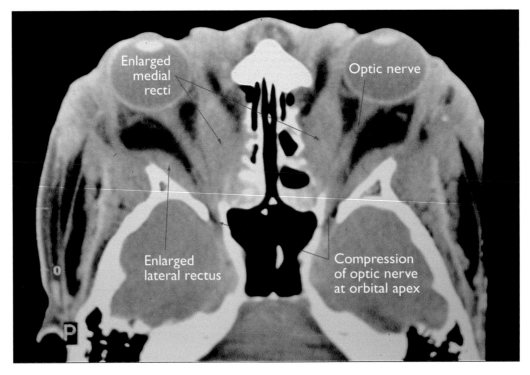

Computerised tomographic scan of head/orbits (transverse section) showing enlarged extraocular muscles and optic nerve compression

Thyroid eye disease may lead to **permanent visual impairment** in two main ways. First, **compression of the optic nerve** by swollen extraocular muscles at the orbital apex and secondly, **severe corneal exposure** and ulceration due to globe **proptosis**. Patients may also have **diplopia** secondary to involvement of extraocular muscles in the inflammatory disease process.

6.15 Blow-Out Fracture of the Orbit

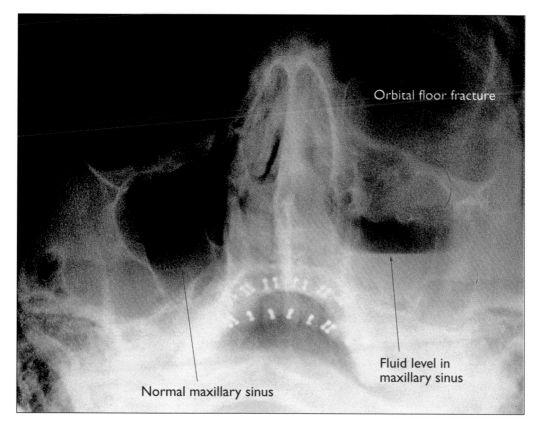

Orbital floor fracture

Fluid level in
maxillary sinus

Normal maxillary sinus

X-ray showing blow-out fracture of the left orbit with fluid in the maxillary sinus

Direct blunt trauma to the globe or orbital rim may produce a fracture of the orbital wall(s).
The **medial wall** and **orbital floor** are the commonest sites of fracture; it may be necessary
to repair the orbital floor. Patients may have **diplopia** if orbital contents are trapped in the
fracture, and **enophthalmos** may be apparent. There may be restricted eye movements on
the affected side, particularly upgaze. Reduced infraorbital sensation is associated with floor
fractures. There may be **co-existing damage to the eye**. All cases need ophthalmic
assessment.

6.16 Dacryocystitis

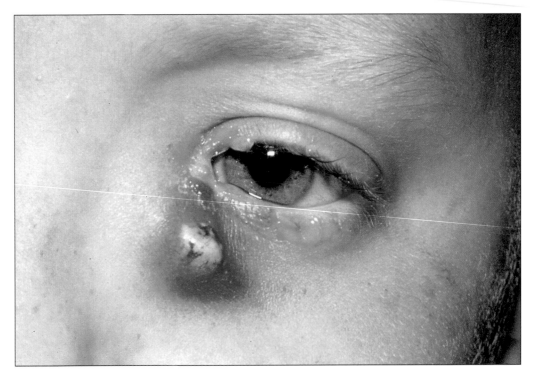

Acute dacryocystitis with purulent discharge and pus in the lacrimal sac pointing through skin

Dacryocystitis is an **acute infection of the lacrimal sac** due to **obstruction** at the level of the **nasolacrimal duct**. Patients present with an extremely painful abscess in the **medial canthal region** which may discharge through the skin. There may be a pre-existing history of a watery eye. Initial treatment is with hot compresses and **systemic antibiotics**, followed usually by lacrimal drainage surgery (**dacryocystorhinostomy** – see 16.22) at a later date.

6.17 Assessment of the Watery Eye – Dacryocystography

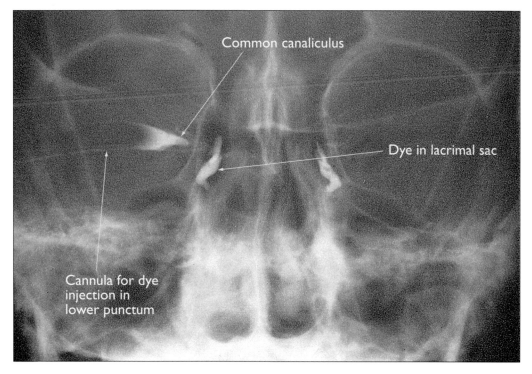

Right dacryocystogram showing dye in the lacrimal system; the completed, left dacryocystogram shows residual dye in the lacrimal sac

Symptoms of **epiphora** (watery eye) are common. When an obstruction in the **nasolacrimal drainage system** is suspected, one can perform **dacryocystography** (DCG) to identify the site of obstruction, and plan surgical intervention. A **radio-opaque dye** is injected into the canaliculi and outlines the anatomy of the upper, lower and common canaliculi, lacrimal sac and nasolacrimal duct.

6.18 Dry Eye – Schirmer's Test

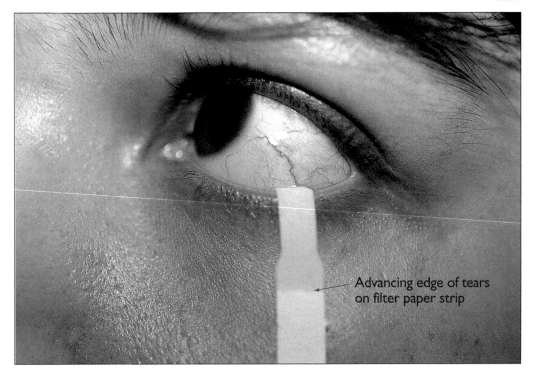

Advancing edge of tears on filter paper strip

Patient undergoing Schirmer's test. A strip of filter paper has been folded into the fornix

Dry eye syndromes are extremely common and are a source of severe ocular discomfort in many patients. Causes include **lacrimal gland** problems, for example, involutional change, connective tissue disease and sarcoidosis; and **cicatricial disease** of the **conjunctiva**, for example, trachoma and pemphigoid. **Schirmer's test** is a simple measure of aqueous tear production involving the use of a small strip of absorbent filter paper. Initial therapy for dry eyes is replacement with **artificial tears**.

7.1 Infective Conjunctivitis – Bacterial

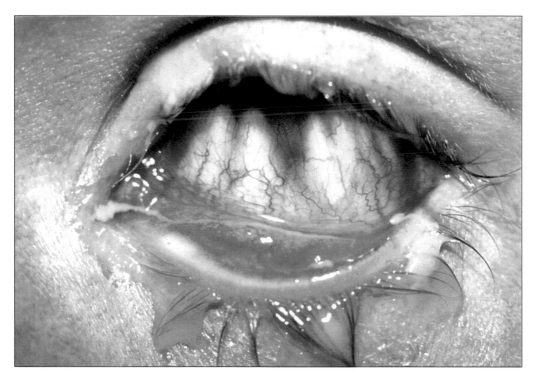

Bacterial conjunctivitis with widespread purulent secretions. The conjunctiva is red but the cornea and pupil reactions are normal

Acute **purulent bacterial conjunctivitis** is an extremely common condition. There is diffuse conjunctival injection and the discharge is often profuse enough to cause the lashes to stick together. When the discharge is washed out of the eyes, the **vision is usually normal**. Treatment is with **topical antibiotics** and regular lid toilet. Most cases should show significant improvement within 5 to 7 days of commencing treatment. If the patient develops recurrent episodes of conjunctivitis, one should look for an underlying cause (such as nasolacrimal system obstruction), or consider other diagnoses.

7.2 Infective Adenoviral Keratoconjunctivitis

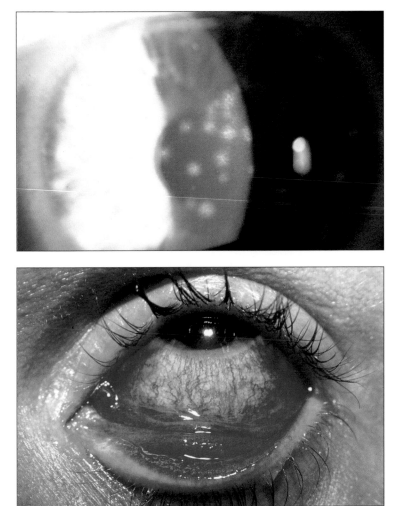

Subepithelial opacities are seen as white dots in the cornea with the microscope

Chronic conjunctivitis caused by persistent adenovirus infection

Patients present with unilateral or bilateral red eyes with a marked **watery discharge**. The patient may have an upper respiratory tract infection and **preauricular lymphadenopathy** is often present. If the patient is **photophobic**, one must suspect **corneal involvement** (keratoconjunctivitis) which is characterised by multiple subepithelial opacities as shown in the illustration. **Visual acuity** can be reduced if the cornea is involved and an ophthalmic referral is suggested. Viral conjunctivitis is highly **contagious** and symptoms can last for up to 6 weeks. Patients should be advised of this. The differential diagnosis for the chronic red eye is very large and is described in **Appendix 2** (see page 173).

7.3 Subtarsal Foreign Body – Upper Lid Eversion

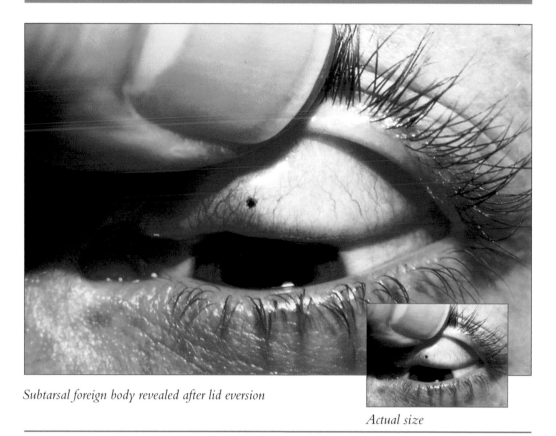

Subtarsal foreign body revealed after lid eversion

Actual size

Patients with a **subtarsal foreign body** can often **localise the gritty sensation** to the area beneath the upper lid. Subtarsal foreign bodies will not be detected unless the upper lid is everted. Prior to everting the upper lid it is helpful to instill a drop of **local anaesthetic** into the eye. The patient is then asked to **look down** to relax the upper lid levator muscle, the lashes of the upper lid are grasped and gentle downward traction applied to the lid. A **cotton-tipped bud** is then placed horizontally against the skin of the lid above the tarsal plate at about 10 mm above lashes, and the lid gently everted. Upper lid eversion should **not** be attempted if a penetrating eye injury is suspected (see 7.5).

7.4 Corneal Foreign Body

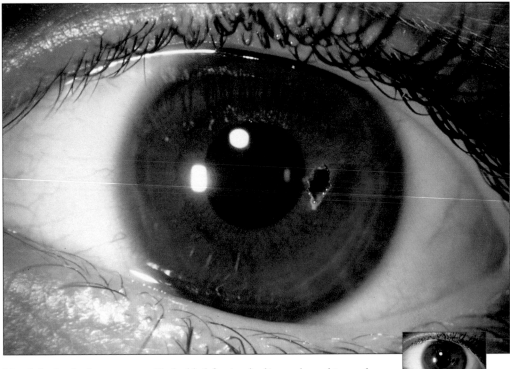

Metal foreign body on cornea. Embedded foreign bodies such as this need removal under local anaesthetic

Actual size

Patients with a **corneal foreign body** (CFB) have an **intensely painful gritty sensation** in the affected eye with marked photophobia and lacrimation. Symptoms may develop several hours after the injury. After instillation of one drop of a **local anaesthetic** agent, for example, Amethocaine 1%, the symptoms are usually temporarily alleviated and examination with a pen torch and magnification will reveal the CFB. The history of the injury is very important; CFBs are common in manual workers. The possibility of a **penetrating eye injury** (see 7.5) and **intraocular foreign body** should be considered in all patients who have been exposed to a **high velocity projectile**, for example, when hammering or chiselling. These patients should have an X-ray of the orbits. Referral is usually necessary for CFB and rust ring removal. The metallic remnants of the foreign body may be deeply embedded in the cornea and may require several visits for complete removal.

7.5 Penetrating Eye Injury

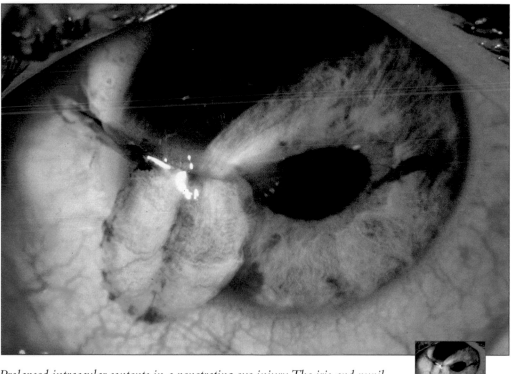

Prolapsed intraocular contents in a penetrating eye injury. The iris and pupil are abnormal and distorted

Actual size

Penetrating eye injuries can result from a wide variety of circumstances and a **detailed history** is essential. Any ocular trauma involving **glass** should raise suspicion. Penetrating eye injuries are often associated with **prolapse of intraocular contents**, for example, the iris. With modern microsurgical techniques it is often possible to repair these severely damaged eyes and restore good vision (see 16.23). It is therefore essential to **prevent any further damage** to the eye when the patient is first seen. Care should be taken to **avoid applying any pressure** to the lids or globe, and a **rigid shield** should be placed over the eye. Antiemetic therapy should be given if the patient is vomiting. **Urgent (same day)** ophthalmic referral is needed.

7.6 Chemical Eye Injury

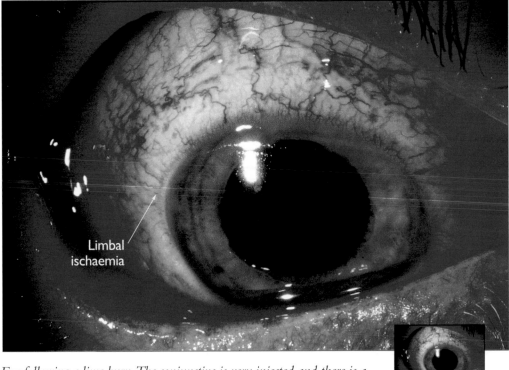

Limbal
ischaemia

Eye following a lime burn. The conjunctiva is very injected and there is a limbal whitening due to capillary shutdown

Actual size

Chemical eye injuries represent an **absolute emergency**. Unless **immediate copious irrigation** of the eyes occurs then the patient may suffer irreversible loss of vision. **Alkaline agents** are the most destructive. Whatever the chemical agent, irrigation with a large volume of **water** or normal saline should be commenced and continued for **at least 10 minutes**. This irrigation should take priority and should be performed before attempting to contact an ophthalmologist. Irrigation should continue until the **pH** of the fluid irrigated from the eye is **consistently neutral**. It is especially important to remove large pieces of particulate matter, for example lime, which may be hidden in the fornices (lid eversion is necessary). **Urgent** transfer to an ophthalmic unit is then necessary.

7.7 Traumatic Hyphaema

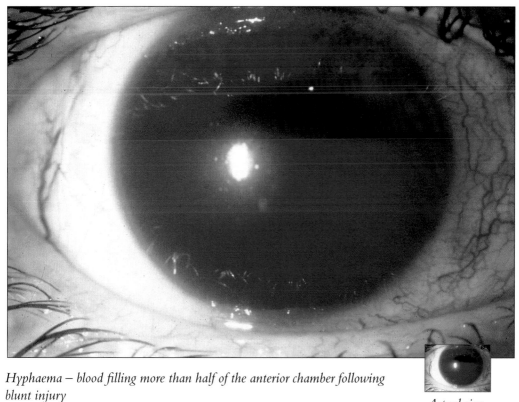

Hyphaema – blood filling more than half of the anterior chamber following blunt injury

Actual size

Traumatic hyphaema usually results from **blunt trauma** to the globe or orbit, for example, from a tennis ball injury. The possibility that there could be a co-existing occult globe perforation should be considered. Traumatic hyphaema is often associated with **elevated intraocular pressure** and retinal trauma. Patients need **urgent (same day)** referral and should be advised regarding **strict rest** for a period of about **7 days** and should avoid significant activity (including sexual activity). The principal serious complication to avoid in the first week after a traumatic hyphaema is a **secondary re-bleed**.

7.8 Dendritic Ulcer – Herpes Simplex Keratitis

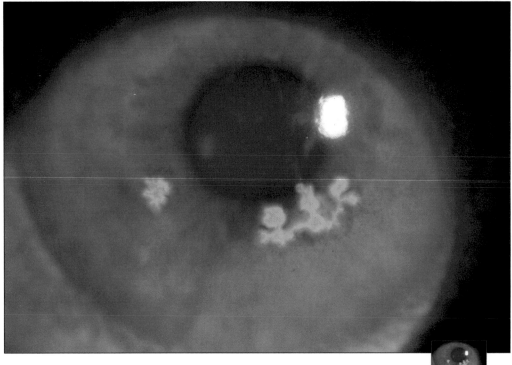

Branching Herpes simplex lesion on cornea stained with fluorescein (yellow stain)

Actual size

Herpetic infections of the cornea are common and recurrent episodes of inflammation can lead to severe corneal scarring. The patient may have a previous history of herpetic disease elsewhere, for example, **'cold sores'** on the lips or eyelids. **Corneal lesions** are characteristically **dendritic** (branching) and stain with **fluorescein** and rose bengal. Reduced corneal sensitivity is often present. It is important to initiate prompt topical **antiviral** therapy.

7.9 Geographical Corneal Ulcer – Inappropriate Steroid Use

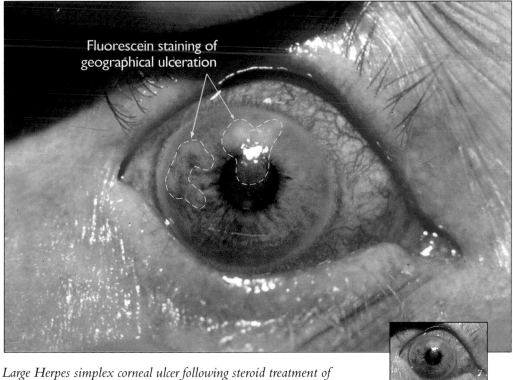

Fluorescein staining of geographical ulceration

Large Herpes simplex corneal ulcer following steroid treatment of a patient presenting with conjunctivitis

Actual size

If topical steroid medications are given to a patient who has a **Herpes simplex** dendritic ulcer of the cornea, the results can be **devastating**. Uncontrolled viral replication can rapidly lead to the formation of a large **'amoeboid' geographical ulcer** of the cornea – with **permanent visual loss**. Topical steroid treatment should never be prescribed without a definite diagnosis in cases of 'red eye' (see page 173). It is easy to miss the diagnosis of many corneal lesions unless fluorescein drops are instilled into the conjunctival sac. Always remove contact lenses before instilling fluorescein.

7.10 Marginal Keratitis

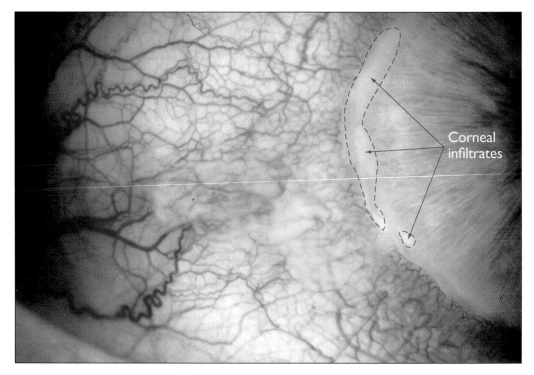

Peripheral corneal inflammatory infiltrates in marginal keratitis

Patients with **marginal keratitis** present with a painful, gritty, photophobic red eye. **Small, white, sterile inflammatory infiltrates** are visible in the **peripheral cornea**. Patients often have co-existing lid margin disease (**blepharitis** – see 6.8 or rosacea). It is often difficult to differentiate marginal keratitis from an infective corneal ulcer, and **immediate** ophthalmic attention is necessary.

7.11 Contact Lens-related Keratitis

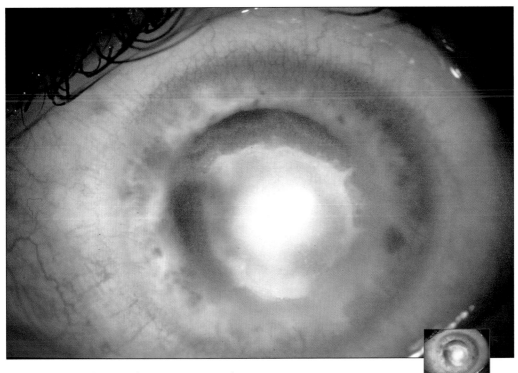

Corneal abscess due to infection in a contact lens wearer

Actual size

There are many causes of inflammatory corneal disease associated with contact lens wear. The most serious problem is a **contact lens-related infection**. Patients often present with a painful, photophobic red eye and are unable to wear their contact lenses. A discrete **corneal abscess** may be visible. Many organisms can cause corneal infection including **Acanthamoebal** species present in domestic tap water. **Immediate** ophthalmic referral is essential because certain organisms such as pseudomonas or pneumococcus can cause irreversible damage to the eye within 24 hours if left untreated. Contact lens wearers should not use their contact lenses if they have a red eye or discharge.

7.12 Allergic Conjunctivitis — Giant Papillae

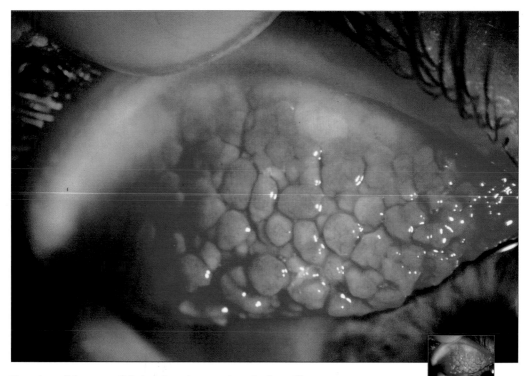

Eversion of the upper lid showing giant conjunctival papillae

Actual size

There is a strong association between chronic allergic eye disease and **atopy. Severe itching** and the presence of a **chronic stringy, mucoid discharge** are prominent features. When the upper lids are everted, the tarsal conjunctiva is often red and oedematous with numerous **giant papillae. Allergen avoidance**, for example, house dust mite, is an important part of therapy. Agents that **stabilise mast cells** and reduce itching are the main forms of treatment and may need to be used on a long-term basis. It may be necessary to use topical steroid drops to control allergic eye disease, but these should **only** be used under very close ophthalmic supervision. Chronic use of topical steroids may result in cataract and glaucoma.

7.13 Pterygium

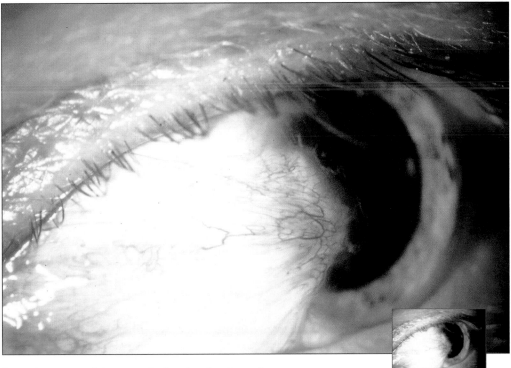

Pterygium encroaching towards the visual axis on the cornea

Actual size

Pterygia are caused by light (actinic) damage and are common in people who have spent long periods in hot climates. They appear as fleshy, vascular growths extending from the conjunctiva onto the cornea, and occur most commonly in the **medial** conjunctival area. They are **often asymptomatic** and need no treatment. They may, however, be associated with marked ocular surface discomfort and may grow towards the visual axis. **Surgical excision** is the treatment of choice for progressive pterygia, but there is a significant **recurrence** rate after surgery.

7.14 Episcleritis

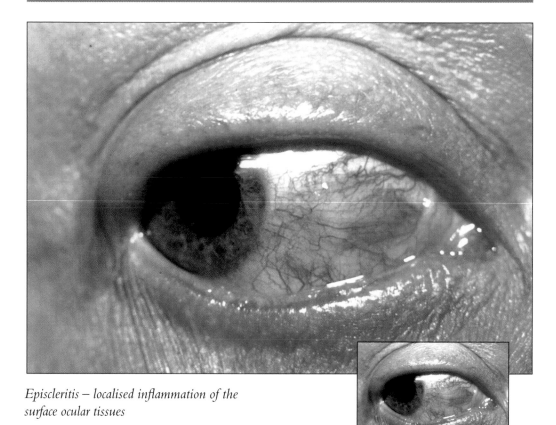

Episcleritis – localised inflammation of the surface ocular tissues

Actual size

Episcleritis is a **self-limiting** and often recurrent, **non-painful, focal inflammation of the episcleral tissues.** The disease tends to affect adults between the ages of 30 and 40, and is not usually associated with systemic disease. Most cases will resolve without treatment, but the application of topical steroids or non-steroidal agents will speed up resolution. It is very important to differentiate episcleritis from scleritis which is a more serious condition (see table opposite).

7.15 Scleritis

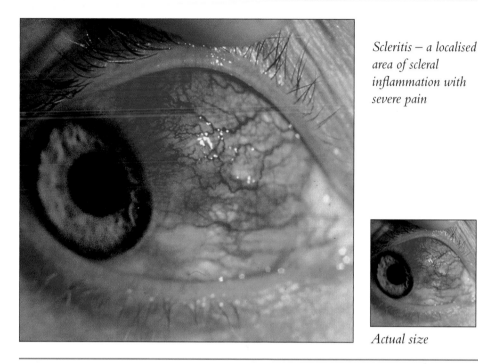

Scleritis – a localised area of scleral inflammation with severe pain

Actual size

Scleritis is a **serious ocular inflammatory disease**, which is often associated with an underlying **systemic collagen vascular disease**, for example, rheumatoid arthritis. Scleritis may also occur as a delayed complication following ocular surgery. Patients complain of a **severe dull ache** in the eye which often prevents them sleeping. The eye may have either a **nodular** or **diffuse dull purple-red area** of **inflammation**. Scleritis requires urgent treatment and medical work-up.

Common Features Distinguishing Episcleritis and Scleritis		
	Episcleritis	Scleritis
Age:	*4th decade – female>male*	*4th – 6th decade - female>male*
Pain:	*Absent or mild discomfort*	*Often severe, dull ache in eye interferes with sleep*
Redness:	*Superficial injection (red) Blanches with topical phenylephrine*	*Deep injection (purple-red) No blanching with phenylephrine*
Vision:	*Usually normal*	*Potential for severe visual loss*
Associated Uveitis:	*Unusual*	*Common*
Systemic Disease:	*Rare*	*Common (e.g. Rheumatoid arthritis)*
Course:	*Often self-limiting*	*May be a protracted course*

7.16 Cicatricial Conjunctivitis – Pemphigoid

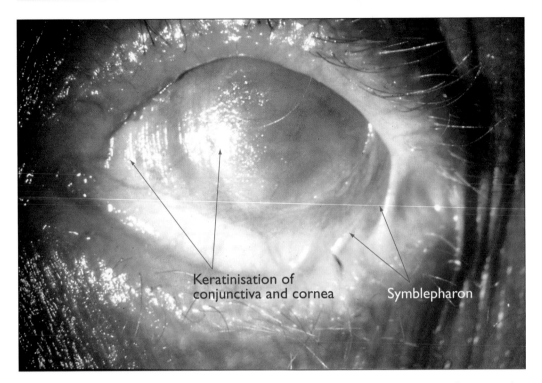

Keratinisation of
conjunctiva and cornea

Symblepharon

Ocular cicatricial pemphigoid – severe scarring of lid and conjunctival tissue with secondary corneal opacification

In **cicatricial conjunctivitis**, for example, in pemphigoid, the predominant feature is the presence of **chronic conjunctival inflammation**, with the formation of marked scarring including adhesions between the conjunctiva of the globe and the lid **(symblepharon)**. In late disease there is a marked **dry eye syndrome** (see 6.18), **lid malpositions** (see 6.3) and **corneal scarring**. If the disease is diagnosed at an early stage then **immunosuppressive therapy** can improve the visual prognosis.

7.17 Scleromalacia Perforans

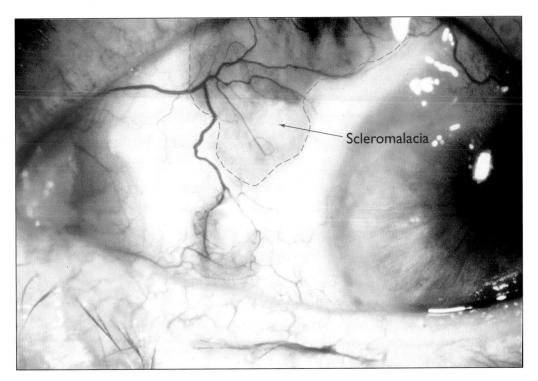

Scleromalacia

Scleromalacia (thin sclera) resulting from previous scleral inflammation

Some severe ocular inflammatory diseases, for example, scleritis in association with rheumatoid arthritis can lead to **massive scleral thinning** (scleromalacia). High dose systemic immunosuppressive therapy may be needed to **prevent extensive scleral destruction** and perforation of the globe.

7.18 Subconjunctival Haemorrhage

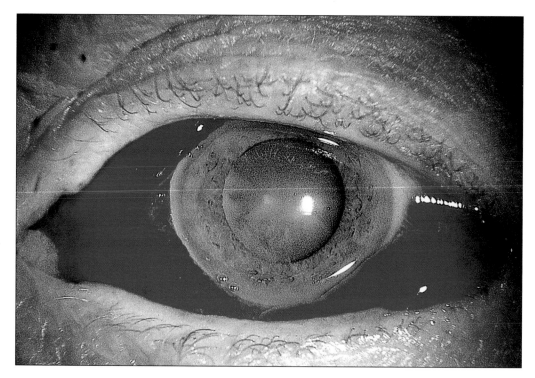

Diffuse subconjunctival haemorrhage (note the co-existing cataract)

Patients are often alarmed when they have a **subconjunctival haemorrhage** due to the dramatic appearance of the anterior segment. The diffuse red haemorrhage leads to the loss of all conjunctival and episcleral detail. It is important to check the patient's **blood pressure** and exclude an underlying **bleeding diathesis**, but no cause is found in most patients. If a patient has **recurrent** subconjunctival haemorrhages, one should consider the possibility of an **orbital vascular anomaly**. If there is a subconjunctival haemorrhage associated with trauma, one must suspect a penetrating eye injury (see 7.5).

8.1 Acute Angle-Closure Glaucoma

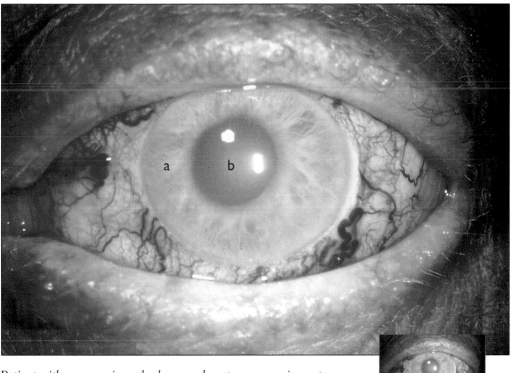

Patient with severe pain and a hazy, oedematous cornea in acute angle-closure glaucoma. (a) Hazy cornea. (b) Fixed, vertically oval, mid-dilated pupil

Actual size

Patients with acute angle-closure glaucoma (AACG) present with severe ocular and periorbital pain and reduced vision in the affected eye(s). Patients may be vomiting and usually feel extremely unwell. The eye on the side with AACG is often injected, with a hazy oedematous cornea and a vertically oval, non-reactive, mid-dilated pupil. A history of prodromal subacute attacks of angle-closure may be present with intermittent episodes of red painful eyes or of seeing haloes around bright lights. After an abortive attack (which may settle overnight), there may be minimal residual signs of the episode. Therefore, an accurate history is essential. Symptoms may be exacerbated by reading, reduced levels of illumination or emotional episodes. People, particularly women, with hypermetropia (see 5.2) are at an increased risk of developing AACG. Urgent (same day) ophthalmic referral is essential.

8.2 Gonioscopy – Open Angle Glaucoma

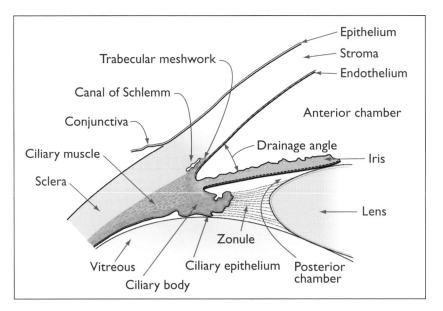

Cross-section of the drainage angle

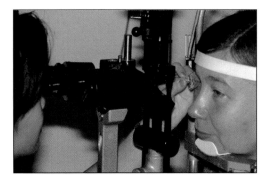

Gonioscopy examination using slit lamp
microscope and contact lens

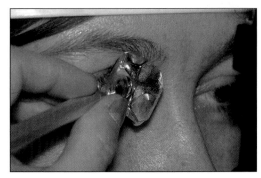

Gonioscopy – close-up of contact lens applied
to eye

Gonioscopy is a technique which enables the ophthalmologist to examine the **drainage angle** of the eye, by using a specially designed **contact lens**. Patients with **glaucoma** can be grouped into two broad categories on the basis of this examination: **open angle** glaucoma and **closed angle** glaucoma, depending on whether the drainage angle structures are visible or not. The distinction between open and closed angle glaucoma is critical because both treatment and prognosis are different in the two groups. **Primary open angle glaucoma** (POAG) is the most common form of glaucoma in the western world, and affects about 2% of the population over the age of 60.

8.3 YAG Laser Peripheral Iridotomy

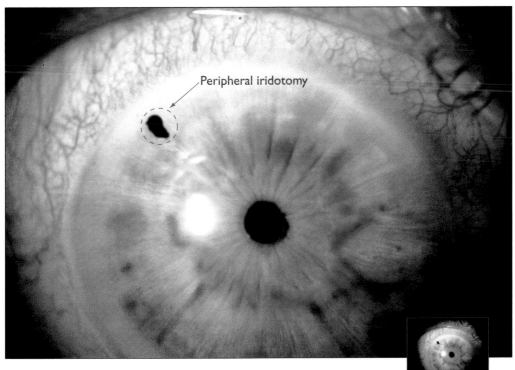

Peripheral iridotomy

Appearance of a superior peripheral iridotomy after YAG laser treatment

Actual size

In cases of acute or chronic **angle-closure glaucoma** (see 8.1), relative **pupil-block** can often be alleviated by creating a **full thickness hole** through the peripheral iris, a procedure called **peripheral iridotomy** (PI). This procedure can be performed as an **out-patient** with the photodisruptive YAG laser which vaporises tissue. The procedure may also be performed **prophylactically** in eyes **at risk** of angle-closure, for example, **high hypermetropes** (see 5.2).

8.4 Normal Optic Disc

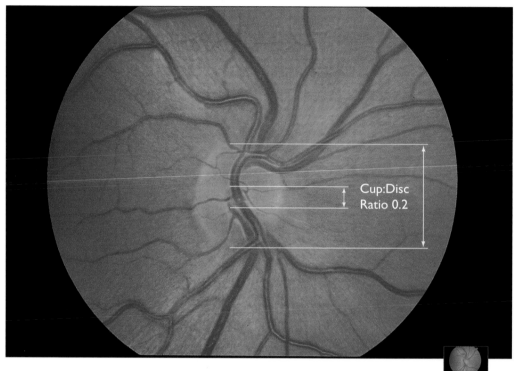

Cup:Disc Ratio 0.2

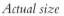

Normal optic disc with a vertical cup:disc ratio of 0.2

Actual size

The spectrum of appearance of normal optic discs is very large, but certain features can help to distinguish a normal disc. The neural rim tissue should be **pink** and **clearly defined**. There is often a high degree of **symmetry** between the disc morphology in the two eyes, particularly with reference to the **vertical cup:disc ratio** (c/d ratio). A large percentage of the population have a c/d ratio of 0.5 or less. Studies have shown that if one has a c/d ratio of 0.6 or greater, or a difference in c/d ratio of greater than 0.2 between the two eyes, then there is a significant risk of developing glaucoma.

8.5 Glaucomatous Cupping of the Optic Disc

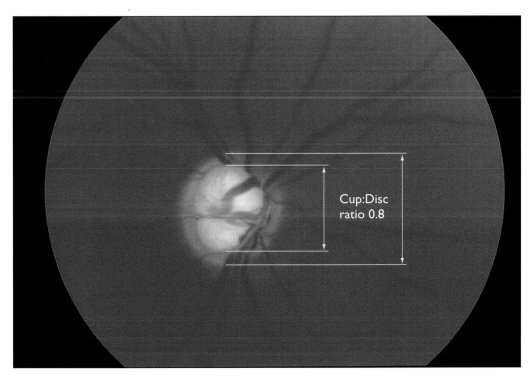

Cup:Disc
ratio 0.8

*Glaucomatous optic disc – pallor, neuroretinal rim thinning, nasal displacement of vessels
and a vertical cup:disc ratio of 0.8*

The classical feature of damage to the optic nerve in glaucoma is cupping. The most important risk factor for the development of optic disc cupping is elevated intraocular pressure. Reduced blood flow to the optic nerve head is also thought to be a factor in some patients. In glaucomatous cupping the amount of pink, healthy neural rim tissue is decreased resulting in an increased cup:disc ratio (usually measured in the vertical plane). Diffuse neural tissue loss results in a concentrically enlarged cup, but focal neural loss may also occur resulting in a focal notch in the neural rim. If there is asymmetrical optic disc cupping or marked pallor of the discs, one should consider the possibility of glaucoma. Splinter haemorrhage(s) on the disc indicate the site of future nerve fibre layer damage.

8.6 Glaucomatous Visual Field Defect

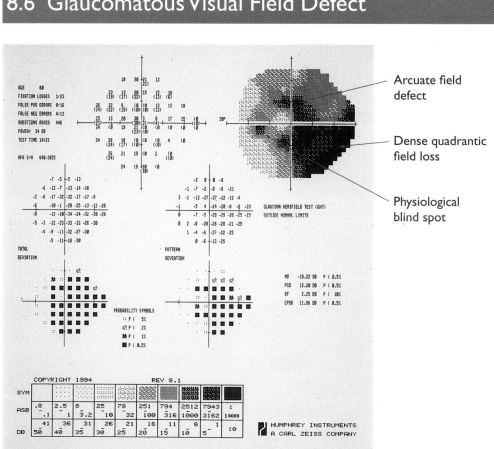

Arcuate field defect

Dense quadrantic field loss

Physiological blind spot

Computerised printout showing advanced glaucomatous visual field defect

Automated visual fields provide an excellent technique for **sequentially** assessing the degree of glaucomatous visual field loss in a patient. Automated fields are **tiring** for the patient and require a **high degree of concentration** and, therefore, are not appropriate for all patients. Classical glaucomatous **arcuate scotomas**, **nasal steps** and **paracentral scotomas** in the central 24 to 30 degrees of the visual field are readily identified. Even with sophisticated automated perimetry, it is estimated that about **30 to 50%** of the fibres in the optic nerve must be damaged before a reproducible visual field defect becomes apparent.

8.7 Normal (Low) Tension Glaucoma

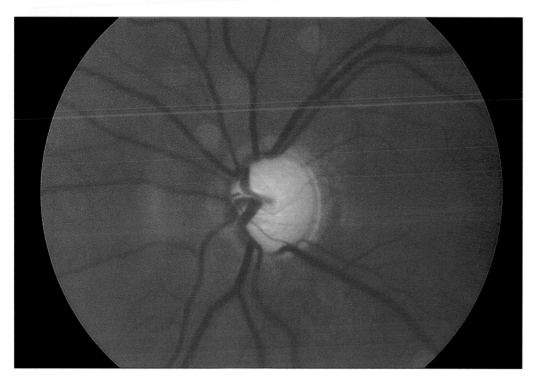

Severe pathological optic disc cupping (cup:disc ratio >0.9) with almost total neuroretinal rim loss

In this form of open angle glaucoma, the classical features of cupping of the optic nerve head (see 8.5) are seen in the absence of statistically elevated intraocular pressure (IOP). Normal (low) tension glaucoma (NTG) may be associated with vasospastic diseases such as migraine and Raynaud's phenomenon, and there may be a history of a previous hypotensive episode or blood loss. Patients often require IOP phasing, in which multiple IOP measurements are made throughout the day, to exclude undetected spikes of raised IOP. Management is initially aimed at lowering the IOP since there is now evidence that lower IOP correlates with improved visual function in progressive diseases. Occasionally one can see features of NTG in patients with a compressive lesion (see 3.4) of the anterior visual pathway, and this possibility should be considered with those patients whose history and examination findings are suspicious, or when the pattern of disease progression is atypical.

8.8 Neovascular Glaucoma

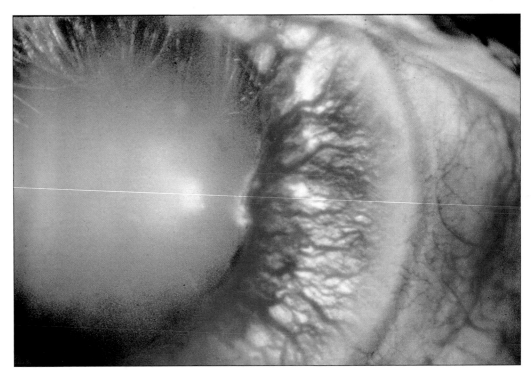

Rubeosis iridis – new vessels on iris, fixed pupil and cataract

Neovascular glaucoma has many causes, but the mechanism common to all is the production of **angiogenic growth factors** from **ischaemic retina**. New **abnormal blood vessels** invade the **drainage angle** of the eye (see 8.2) causing severe intractable secondary glaucoma, often with **very high intraocular pressure** and **corneal oedema**. Abnormal vessels may be visible on the iris **(rubeosis iridis)**.

Diseases associated with Neovascular Glaucoma	
Central retinal venous occlusion	11.3
Proliferative diabetic retinopathy	11.7
Arterial occlusion	11.4
Intraocular tumours	12.1
Intraocular inflammatory disease	9.2

9.1 Uveitis – Juvenile Chronic Arthritis

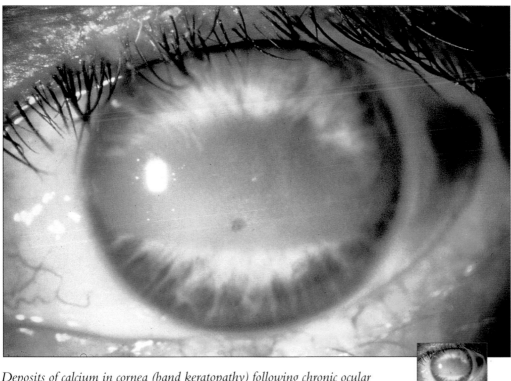

Deposits of calcium in cornea (band keratopathy) following chronic ocular inflammation

Actual size

Juvenile chronic arthritis (JCA) is a polyarthropathy/systemic disease, certain forms of which are associated with a **chronic, non-granulomatous anterior uveitis**. Of the children that develop uveitis, about 25% will be at risk of severe **vision-threatening** complications, particularly in those with arthritis in less than five joints (pauciarticular). The onset of ocular inflammatory disease is usually **asymptomatic** and therefore it is necessary to **screen** children at risk of developing complications. The main ocular complications are severe secondary **glaucoma**, **cataract** and **band keratopathy**.

9.2 Anterior Uveitis – Keratic Precipitates

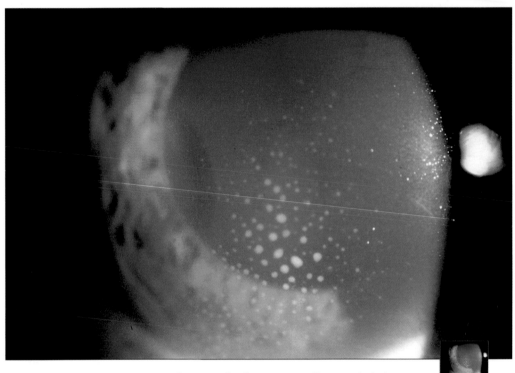

'Mutton fat' keratic precipitates – deposits of inflammatory cells on endothelium   *Actual size*

During an attack of acute anterior uveitis (AAU) there is usually a dull ocular/periorbital pain, photophobia, and a mild reduction in vision. The condition is often unilateral, but both eyes can be affected simultaneously. There is circumcorneal 'ciliary' injection (redness is more prominent overlying the inflamed ciliary body) and a hypopyon (see 9.4) may be present. When the anterior segment of the eye is examined with a **slit-lamp biomicroscope**, one may see inflammatory cells, flare (increased scattering of light through aqueous with a high protein content), fibrin and **cellular deposits** on the corneal endothelium – **keratic precipitates** (KPs). The morphology of the KPs may give a clue to the aetiology of the uveitis. Large KPs which look like 'mutton fat' are seen in **sarcoidosis**.

9.3 Anterior Uveitis – Posterior Synechiae

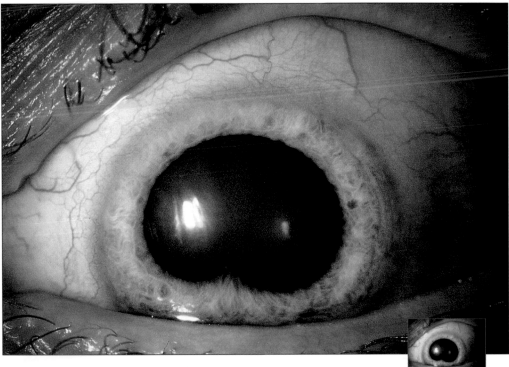

Inferior posterior synechiae at "6 o'clock" position

Actual size

The inflammation in acute anterior uveitis (AAU) is often **recurrent**, but there may be clues that there has been **previous intraocular inflammation** such as **posterior synechiae** which are adhesions between the iris and the anterior surface of the lens. Prompt aggressive treatment of AAU, including dilating drops to mobilise the pupil, helps to prevent the development of posterior synechiae. Severe 360 degree posterior synechiae at the pupil margin can obstruct aqueous flow, and cause **pupil block glaucoma**

9.4 Hypopyon Uveitis

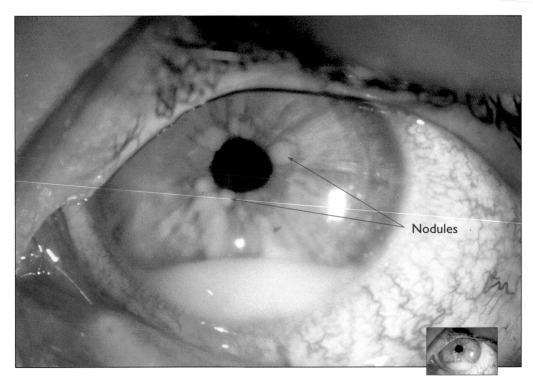

Nodules

Hypopyon with Koeppe & Busacca nodules   *Actual size*

The observation of a settled level of white inflammatory material in the inferior anterior chamber (hypopyon) is an important sign – representing the presence of either a **severe inflammatory or infective process**. Inflammatory ocular diseases associated with an hypopyon include **Behçet's disease**, **sarcoidosis** and **ankylosing spondylitis**. Infective causes include corneal abscess, post–operative endophthalmitis and metastatic endophthalmitis. The presence of an hypopyon means that an **immediate** ophthalmic opinion is required, especially if there is any chance of an infective aetiology, for example, post-operatively.

9.5 Oral Ulceration – Behçet's Disease

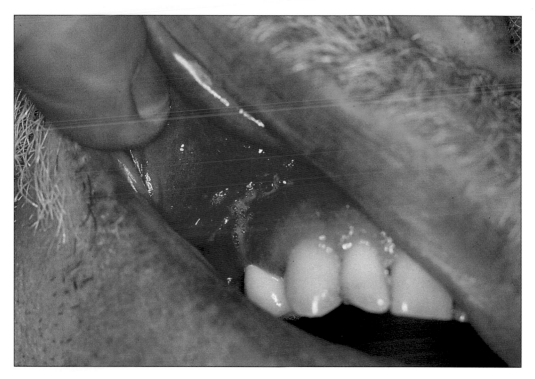

Oral ulceration can occur anywhere in the mouth

It is important to perform a full **systemic enquiry** in cases of **uveitis**, in order to identify those patients who have an **associated systemic disease**. Oral and genital ulceration may occur in syphilis or **Behçet's disease**. Cervical, lumbar and sacroiliac joint pain may suggest **ankylosing spondylitis**. The patient may have the skin lesions of **psoriasis**, or pulmonary symptoms which may be from underlying **sarcoidosis** or **tuberculosis**. The patient may have a history of **inflammatory bowel disease**, or have **diabetes mellitus**. Although many cases are **idiopathic**, there are a wide range of systemic diseases which can be found in association with uveitis.

9.6 AIDS – Cytomegalovirus Retinitis

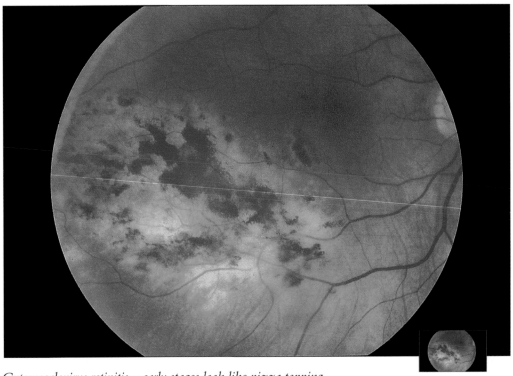

Cytomegalovirus retinitis – early stages look like pizza topping

Actual size

Cytomegalovirus (CMV) causes an opportunistic **retinal infection (retinitis)** in patients with the acquired immunodeficiency syndrome **(AIDS)**. The retinal lesions appear as white areas of retinitis with associated haemorrhage, often occurring along the vascular arcades at the posterior pole. The drugs used for treatment are extremely **toxic** and need close supervision in specialised units. Recent advances include the development of slow–release drug delivery implants which can be placed within the posterior segment of the eye. The incidence of CMV has reduced since the introduction of protease inhibitors.

10.1 Mature Cataract

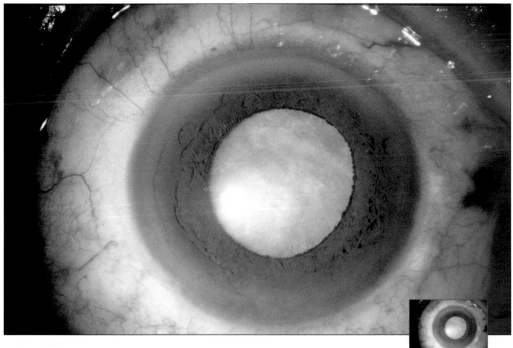

Liquid end-stage mature white cataract

Actual size

Progressive opacification of the crystalline lens in the elderly causes a steady reduction in visual function. In a mature cataract, the level of visual acuity may reduce to hand movements or the perception of light. The absence of a relative afferent pupil defect, a normal **ultrasound** scan (see 4.12) and normal electrodiagnostic testing (see 4.13) can help to exclude significant posterior segment problems prior to planned surgical rehabilitation. Technological advances allow surgeons to remove cataracts at any time before they reach this stage (see 16.6).

10.2 Nuclear Sclerotic Cataract

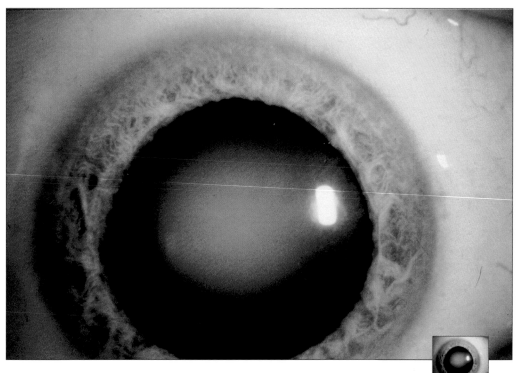

Nuclear sclerosis – opacity in centre of lens

Actual size

A common **aging** change in the lens is the development of progressive **nuclear sclerosis**. In this process the central nuclear core of the lens undergoes **biochemical** and **structural changes** which result in it acquiring a **yellow** and then brown (brunescent) colour. Patients often develop increasing **myopia** as the lens changes and notice that their reading vision improves, often without glasses.

10 The Lens

10.3 Cortical Lens Opacity

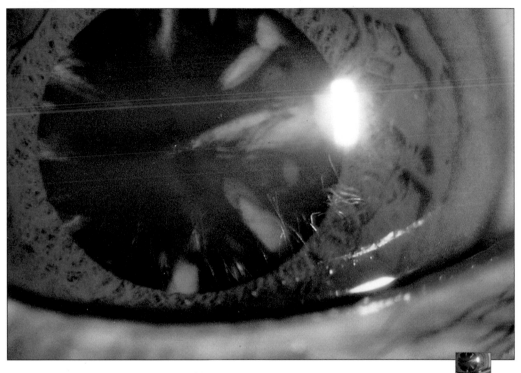

Cortical lens opacities in periphery of lens

Actual size

When the outer cortical part of the lens develops a cataract, this is seen as radiating cortical **spoke-like** opacities. Patients often complain of **distortion** of vision and may experience marked **glare**. The decision about when to offer **cataract surgery** (see 16.5 and 16.6) to a patient is a complex one, and must take into account the **visual requirements** of the patient, the degree of **visual impairment**, the condition of the **fellow eye** and the **risk-benefit ratio** of the operation.

10.4 Posterior Subcapsular Lens Opacity – Red Reflex

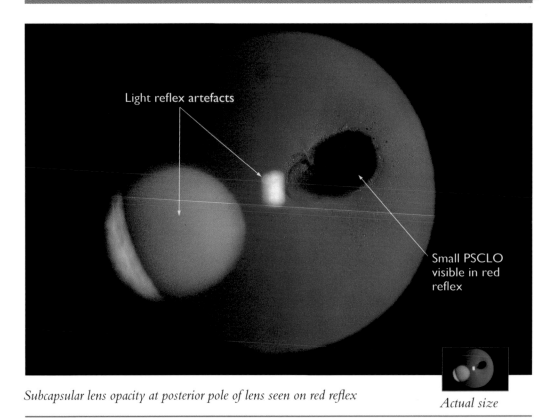

Light reflex artefacts

Small PSCLO visible in red reflex

Subcapsular lens opacity at posterior pole of lens seen on red reflex

Actual size

Even a small amount of **posterior subcapsular lens opacity** (PSCLO) can lead to a marked reduction in visual function, because the opacity is close to the centrally placed nodal point of the eye through which most light rays pass. The effects on vision are particularly apparent when the pupil is **constricted** (miosed), for example, in conditions of bright sunlight. This type of lens opacity is associated with local, topical and systemic **steroid** therapy. An oral dose of Prednisolone greater than 10 mg/day for over one year may produce characteristic PSCLO. When the red reflex is examined with a direct ophthalmoscope (see 4.7) the PSCLO is seen as a dense **central black dot** against the red reflex.

10.5 Ectopia Lentis

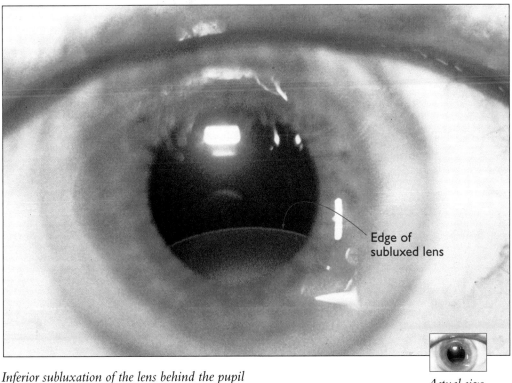

Edge of
subluxed lens

Inferior subluxation of the lens behind the pupil

Actual size

Ectopia lentis refers to the condition in which there is **subluxation/dislocation** of the crystalline lens from the normal position. Lens subluxation is most commonly associated with age, trauma and myopia. Ectopia lentis is a frequent finding in **Marfan's syndrome** (lens usually subluxed upwards), but is also seen in **homocystinuria** (lens usually subluxed downwards), aniridia and the other rare systemic syndromes. Lens dislocation may be associated with **secondary glaucoma** and there is also an increased incidence of **retinal detachment** (see 11.1).

10.6 Traumatic Cataract

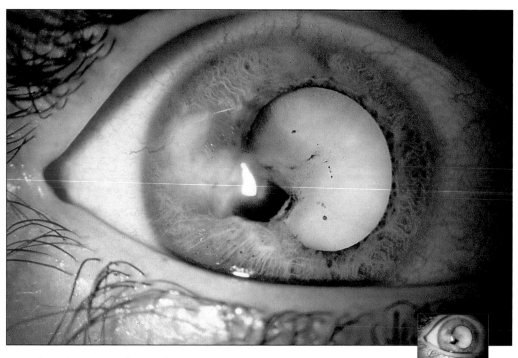

Opacified white lens and corneal scarring after ocular trauma

Actual size

Traumatic cataract can follow both **blunt** and **penetrating ocular trauma**. Surgery to remove the opacified lens can be complicated, especially if the supporting zonular attachments of the lens have been damaged and the lens is subluxed (see 10.5) or unstable. It is not always possible to implant an **intraocular lens** at the time of surgery and other forms of optical correction of aphakia, for example, by contact lens may be necessary.

11 Retinal and Macular Disease

11.1 Retinal Detachment

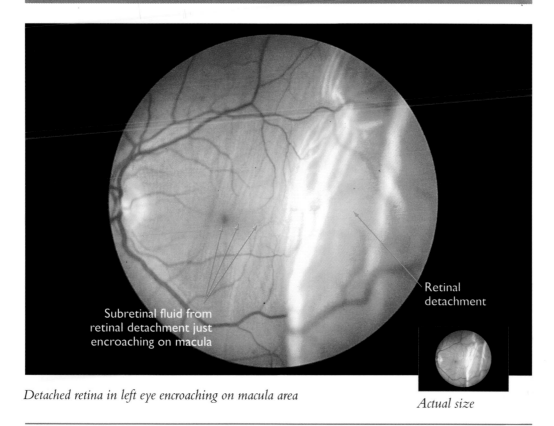

Retinal detachment

Subretinal fluid from retinal detachment just encroaching on macula

Detached retina in left eye encroaching on macula area

Actual size

Patients often present with a short history of **flashes and floaters**. They may also have reduced vision or an advancing visual field defect. Patients with **myopia** (see 5.1) have an increased risk of retinal detachment. **Retinal tears** may occur in patients with an **acute posterior vitreous detachment** (see 11.2), or who have had recent ocular or head trauma. The detached retina often appears pale, elevated and 'corrugated' when compared to surrounding flat retina. **If the retinal detachment is repaired surgically** (see 16.16 and 16.17) *before* the **macula region becomes detached**, the **prognosis is excellent**. Patients should, therefore, be referred for an **urgent (same day)** ophthalmic opinion.

11.2 Posterior Vitreous Detachment

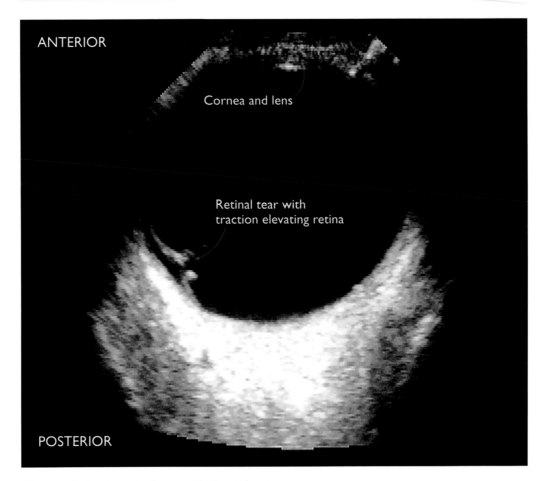

Ultrasound showing retinal tear with elevated retina

In posterior vitreous detachment (PVD), **degenerative** changes in the vitreous body cause the vitreous gel to collapse, clump and exert traction on the retina as shown in the ultrasound above. Patients give a short history of unilateral **flashes**, often in the temporal visual field and an associated **floater**, often described as 'crescent-shaped' or 'like a fly'. If patients develop a visual field defect, one must suspect a secondary **retinal detachment** (see 11.1). All patients with an acute PVD should have a retinal tear excluded by ophthalmic examination and be **warned** of the risk of retinal detachment. Small retinal detachments and retinal tears cannot be seen by direct ophthalmoscopy and require careful ophthalmic examination with scleral indentation (see 4.8) to exclude a small lesion which can progress rapidly.

11.3 Central Retinal Venous Occlusion

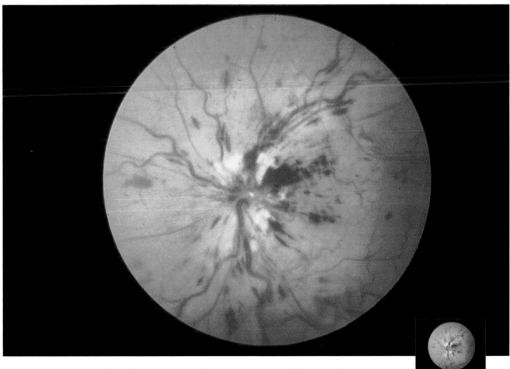

Engorged veins, swollen disc, cotton wool spots and retinal haemorrhages

Actual size

Central retinal venous occlusion (CRVO) presents as **painless acute/subacute loss of vision.** Visual acuity can range from good to very poor. A relative afferent pupil defect (RAPD) may be present. **Retinal haemorrhages** and engorged retinal veins are usually present. Patients should be referred for **urgent** ophthalmic work up to identify and treat patients at risk of neovascular glaucoma (see 8.8). CRVO has a strong association with **hypertension** and other systemic diseases including diabetes mellitus, hypercholesterolaemia and causes of hyperviscosity.

11.4 Central Retinal Artery Occlusion

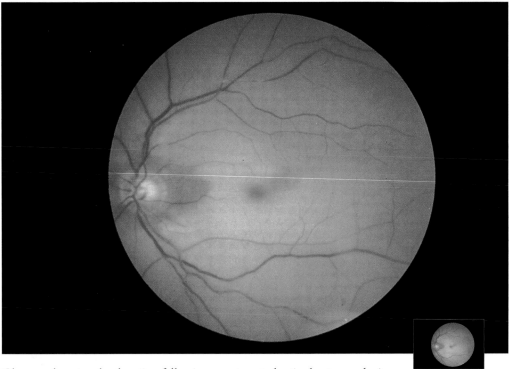

Cherry red spot and pale retina following recent central retinal artery occlusion *Actual size*

Central retinal artery occlusion (CRAO) presents clinically as a **painless, sudden loss of vision**. Patients have very poor vision and a relative afferent pupillary defect. The retina has a **whitened** appearance (due to oedematous ischaemic retina) and the fovea is temporarily seen as a 'cherry red spot'. The presence of a source of emboli, for example, atrial fibrillation and carotid artery disease **must** be sought. It is necessary to exclude giant cell arteritis (see 15.14). **Urgent (same day)** ophthalmic referral is necessary.

11.5 Non-Proliferative Diabetic Retinopathy

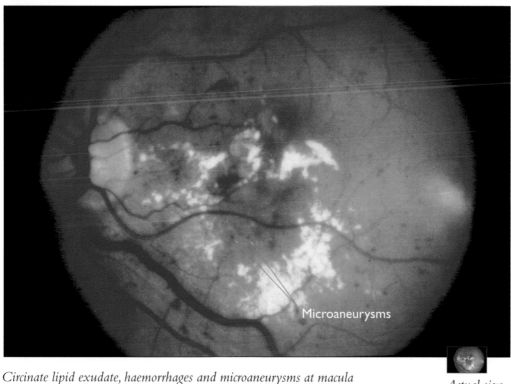

Microaneurysms

Circinate lipid exudate, haemorrhages and microaneurysms at macula

Actual size

Non-proliferative diabetic retinopathy (NPDR) is an initial stage of diabetic retinopathy and varies in severity. Retinal examination may show **microaneurysms, haemorrhage, cotton wool spots, lipid exudate and oedema**. Ophthalmic assessment is necessary in order to detect forms of disease which may progress to significant maculopathy or proliferative disease (see 11.6 and 11.7).

11.6 Exudative Diabetic Maculopathy – Argon Laser Macular Grid

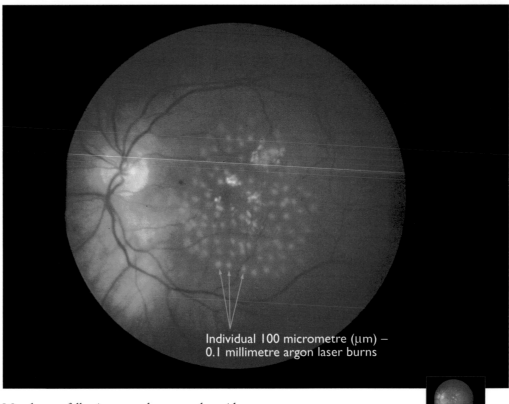

Individual 100 micrometre (µm) –
0.1 millimetre argon laser burns

Macula area following argon laser macular grid

Actual size

In diabetic exudative maculopathy, **leakage of fluid and lipid** into the macula region often results in reduced visual function. In certain cases it is possible to place a **grid** of **100 micrometre** (*µm*) argon laser burns in the macular area, **reducing oedema** and stabilising or improving visual acuity. It is important to manage associated systemic problems such as uncontrolled blood sugar, hypertension and renal failure as they may exacerbate macular oedema.

11.7 Proliferative Diabetic Retinopathy

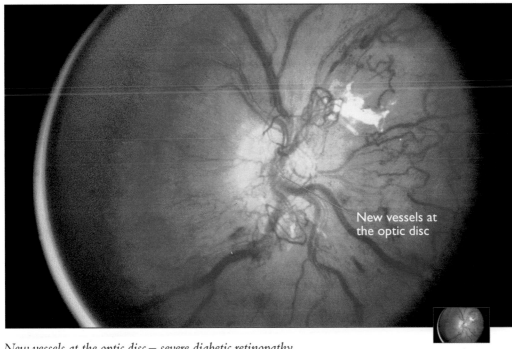

New vessels at
the optic disc

New vessels at the optic disc – severe diabetic retinopathy

Actual size

Proliferative diabetic retinopathy (PDR) is a manifestation of severe diabetic retinopathy in which **new abnormal blood vessels proliferate within the eye**. These are seen as thin tortuous vessels that grow across the retinal surface and into the vitreous cavity. PDR is associated with a high risk of **permanent visual loss** and requires **urgent laser** treatment (see 11.8). PDR is the most common cause of blind registration in the population aged under 55 years. Recent evidence suggests that optimal long-term control of blood sugar is associated with a reduced incidence of blinding diabetic complications.

11.8 Pan-retinal Laser Photocoagulation

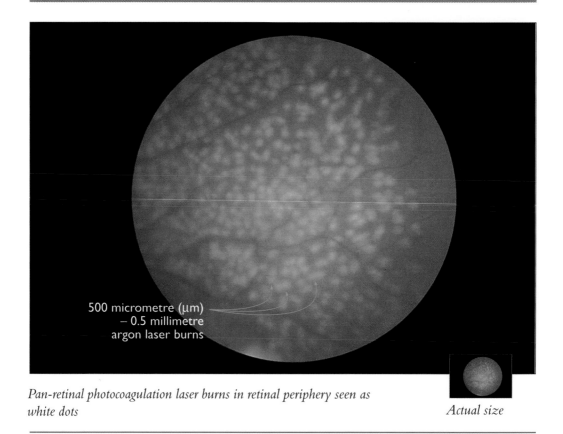

500 micrometre (µm)
– 0.5 millimetre
argon laser burns

Pan-retinal photocoagulation laser burns in retinal periphery seen as
white dots

Actual size

Pan-retinal photocoagulation (PRP) laser treatment is used to **ablate ischaemic retina** and **induce regression** of abnormal new blood vessels in diseases such as proliferative diabetic retinopathy (see 11.7) and central retinal venous occlusion (see 11.3). Retinal burns appear as **white dots** on the retina immediately after treatment and become **pigmented** with time. About 1,500 to 2,500 burns (applied in several treatment sessions) may be needed to induce disease regression.

11.9 Vitreous Haemorrhage

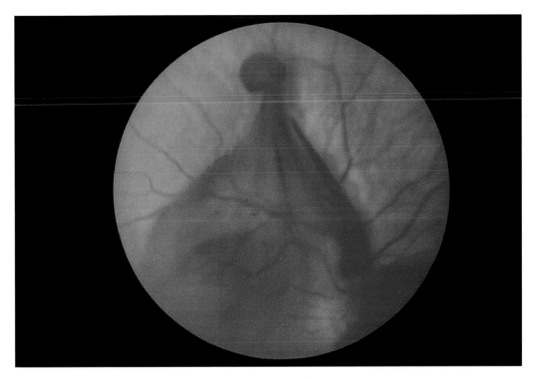

Blood in vitreous obscuring retina – needs careful examination to determine cause

Patients with vitreous haemorrhage often present with **sudden, painless visual loss** in one eye. They may report seeing numerous tiny **floaters** as their vision decreased. Vitreous haemorrhage can occur in association with a large number of diseases including **posterior vitreous detachment** (see 11.2), **trauma, proliferative diabetic retinopathy** (see 11.7), sickle cell retinopathy and central retinal venous occlusion (see 11.3). Vitreous haemorrhage may clear spontaneously over several months, but surgical removal of the blood/vitreous **(vitrectomy)** may be required in persistent haemorrhage or when laser treatment (PRP) to the retina is needed.

11.10 Hypertensive Retinopathy

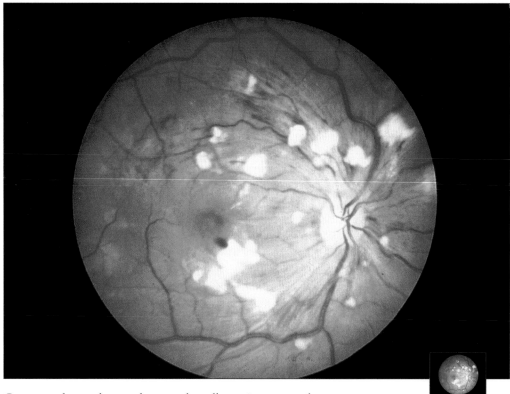

Cotton wool spots, haemorrhages and swollen retina at mucula

Actual size

A spectrum of retinal changes occur in hypertension reflecting the severity and duration of disease. Features include vessel changes such as attenuation and arterio-venous nipping, haemorrhage, cotton wool spots and lipid exudate. If the optic disc is swollen, malignant hypertension should be suspected and treated as a medical emergency. Much useful information can be gained about the systemic vascular condition by examining the retinal blood vessels, and fundal examination should be a routine part of the assessment of all hypertensive patients.

11.11 Age-Related Maculopathy – Drusen

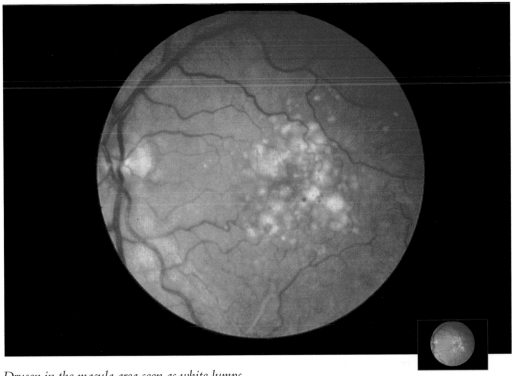

Drusen in the macula area seen as white lumps

Actual size

One of the **aging** changes seen in the macular region is the formation of **drusen**, which are degenerative colloid bodies located between the retinal pigment epithelium and Bruch's membrane. Drusen are seen as **small, yellow-white deposits** in the region of the posterior pole. 'Hard' drusen have sharply defined edges, but 'soft' drusen are often larger, have indistinct edges and may be associated with **exudative maculopathy** (see 11.13).

11.12 Non-Exudative Age-Related Macular Degeneration

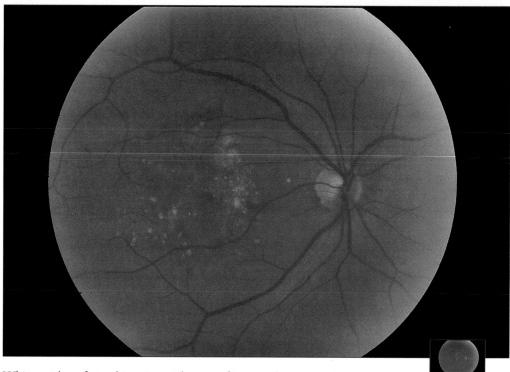

White patches of atrophic retina with areas of increased pigmentation

Actual size

Patients with non–exudative age-related macular degeneration (ARMD) have reduced central visual acuity and may have **metamorphopsia**. Patients often have difficulty **reading** and **recognising faces**. Examination shows a fine pigmentary disturbance and atrophy at the macula. It is important to differentiate **'dry'** (non–exudative) ARMD from exudative ARMD (see 11.13). Patients may benefit from a refraction and assessment for **low visual aids**.

11.13 Exudative Disciform Maculopathy

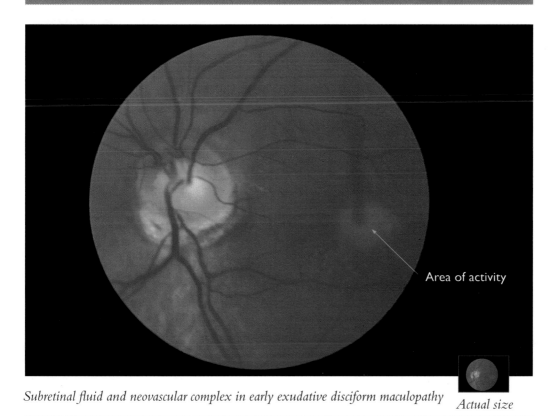

Area of activity

Subretinal fluid and neovascular complex in early exudative disciform maculopathy   *Actual size*

In non-exudative age-related macular degeneration (ARMD), about 30% of patients develop **abnormal new blood vessels** underneath the macula. These vessels leak fluid and blood, which causes the formation of a **sub-retinal scar**. This condition may be associated with **drusen** (see 11.11). The initial subtle symptoms may include **distortion** of vision (metamorphopsia), which can be demonstrated using an **Amsler chart** (see 11.14). Late disease results in dense central visual loss and **functional blindness** (although peripheral vision is retained). All patients with metamorphopsia need **urgent** ophthalmic assessment because **laser photocoagulation** can be used to ablate the abnormal blood vessels in some patients. Signs of disease may be quite subtle and one should place importance on gaining an accurate history of the visual disturbance.

11.14 Amsler Chart

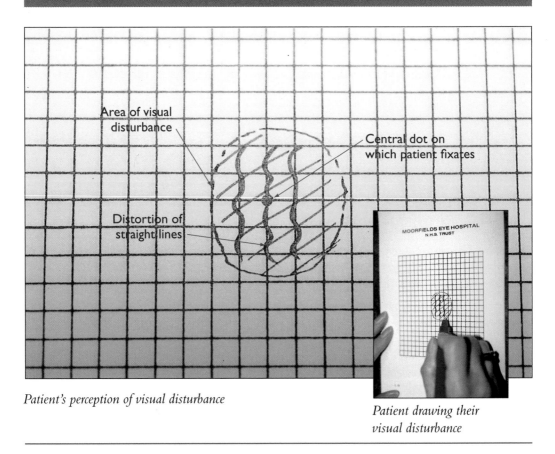

Patient's perception of visual disturbance

Patient drawing their visual disturbance

This is a simple test used to assess patients who have **distortion** of their **central vision** (metamorphopsia). Using the **Amsler Chart**, the patient will see distortion of **straight lines** or will report that some of the central squares are **missing**. The test is a particularly useful means of assessing the good fellow eye of a patient who has severe macular disease in the other eye.

11.15 Retinitis Pigmentosa

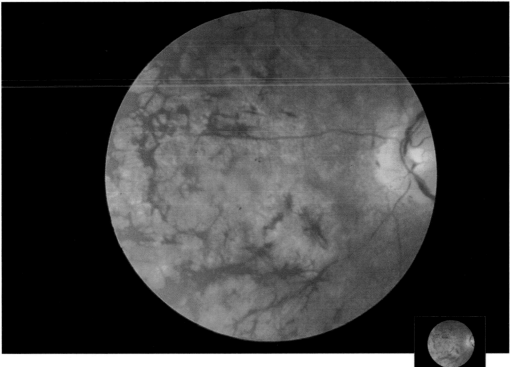

Pigmented retina, attenuated blood vessels and pale disc

Actual size

Retinitis pigmentosa (RP) is an **inherited primary retinal degeneration** and presents with progressive **loss of night vision** and constriction of the peripheral visual field. Findings include spicules of dark **'iron filings'** pigmentation in the retina, arteriolar attenuation and optic disc pallor. The development of associated **cataract** or cystoid macular oedema can reduce central visual function. Patients should be offered **genetic counselling**. Early diagnosis can be facilitated/confirmed by the use of electrodiagnostic testing (see 4.13).

11.16 Choroidal Folds

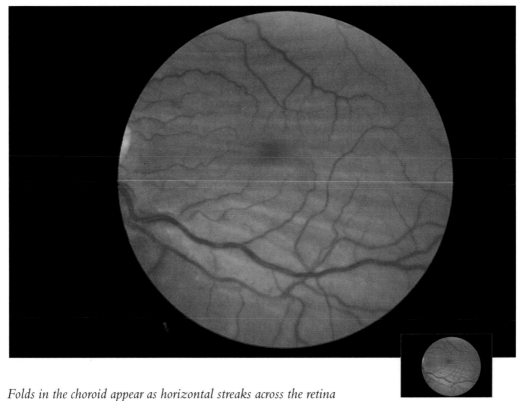

Folds in the choroid appear as horizontal streaks across the retina

Actual size

Choroidal folds at the posterior pole are seen in many diseases including **thyroid eye disease** (see 6.13), **orbital tumours**, posterior **scleritis** (see 7.15) and ocular **hypotony**. Persistent choroidal folds will result in a reduction in visual function.

11.17 Macular Hole

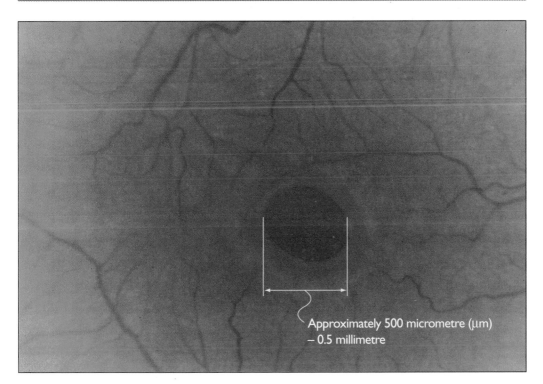

Approximately 500 micrometre (µm) – 0.5 millimetre

Highly magnified picture of a macular hole

Macular holes may be **full or partial thickness**. They may occur as an **idiopathic finding**, possibly related to abnormal vitreo-retinal attachment, or be associated with other ocular inflammatory diseases or trauma. In some cases of full thickness holes, surgical intervention with **vitrectomy** may improve vision. If a patient has a unilateral macular hole, they should **closely monitor** their vision for similar problems with an **Amsler grid** (see 11.14).

11.18 Retinal Trauma – Commotio Retinae

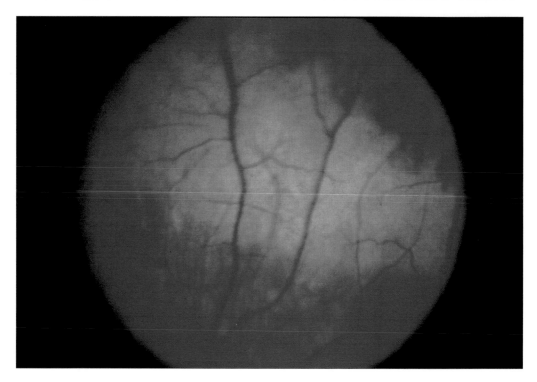

Pale area indicates retinal oedema following blunt trauma

Commotio retinae is the term used to describe retinal oedema seen after **blunt trauma** to the eye. The affected retina has a silvery-white appearance. The presence of commotio retinae is a sign that the eye has suffered a considerable blunt force, and one should look for signs of associated retinal trauma, including retinal haemorrhage and **retinal tears**. Isolated commotio retinae does not require any special treatment.

12 Ocular Oncology

12.1 Choroidal Melanoma

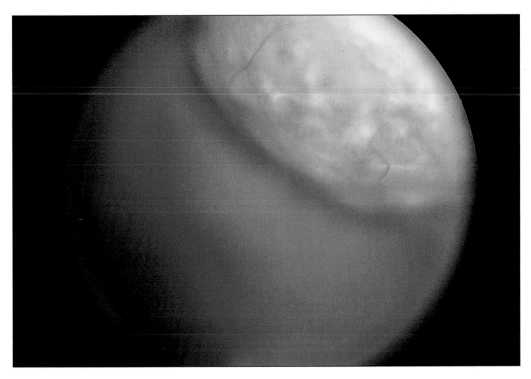

Large raised white/pigmented mass under the retina

Choroidal melanoma is the most common primary **intraocular malignancy**. Patients often present with advanced disease, and late presentation is associated with a **poor prognosis**. Symptoms include reduced visual acuity, advancing visual field defects and flashes and floaters in the affected eye. Treatment options include enucleation (see 16.25), radiotherapy, laser therapy and chemotherapy (often in combination). The **liver** is a common site for delayed metastasis.

12.2 Choroidal Metastatic Deposit

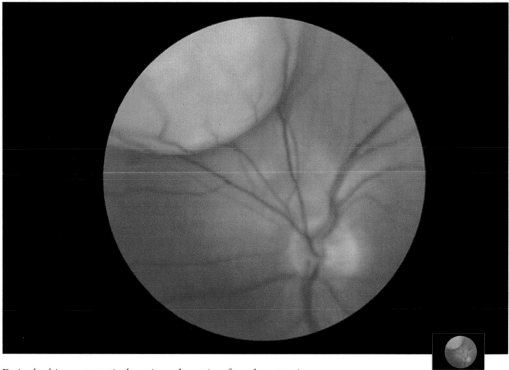

Raised white metastatic deposit under retina from breast primary

Actual size

Secondary metastases usually occur in the region of the **posterior** choroid and usually present with visual loss, flashes, floaters and advancing visual field defects. **Primary tumours** with metastases to the choroid include **breast**, **lung**, thyroid, kidney and testis. Palliative treatment with radiotherapy may be helpful for some patients.

12.3 Choroidal Naevus

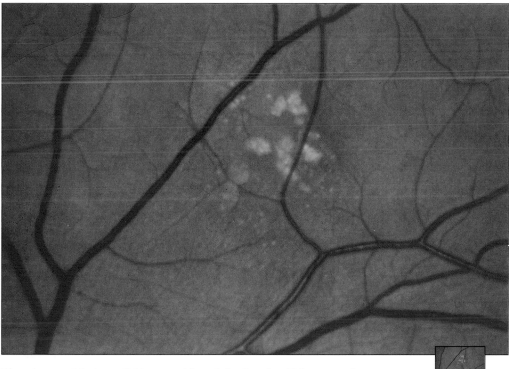

*Flat pigmented lesions of this type although benign should be assessed
in clinic*

Actual size

Choroidal naevi are **benign**, asymptomatic lesions which occur in about 5% of the population and are often found on routine examination. They appear as **flat**, **pigmented** choroidal
lesions about 1 to 2 disc diameters in size. Drusen may occur on the surface of the naevus.
There are varying opinions whether naevi may on occasions undergo **malignant change**.
For this reason, all pigmented fundal lesions should be assessed by an ophthalmologist.

12.4 Iris Melanoma

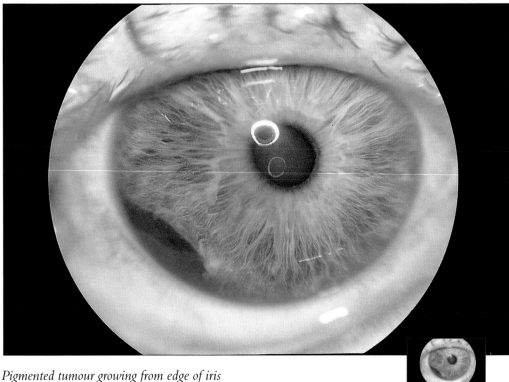

Pigmented tumour growing from edge of iris

Actual size

Pigmented tumours of the iris are **rare**. Patients may report the fact that an existing iris lesion has **increased in size** or has changed **colour**. If the lesion invades the drainage angle of the eye, there may be secondary **glaucoma**. All patients with suspicious iris lesions should have regular ophthalmic assessment and anterior segment **photography**.

13.1 Convergent Strabismus (Esotropia)

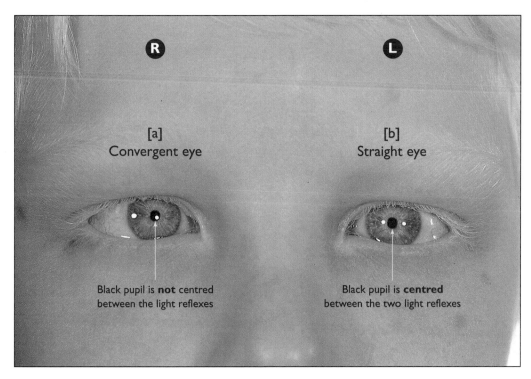

Right convergent strabismus (esotropia) in a child with albinism

Parents report that one or both eyes 'turn in', often when the child is tired. Convergent strabismus is the most common form of strabismus in children and may be idiopathic or associated with hypermetropia (see 5.2) or rarely, other ocular or neurological disease, for example, sixth nerve palsy (see 15.8). The corneal light reflex is temporal to the pupil on the convergent eye (see illustration above [a]), and centred on the pupil in the straight fixing eye [b]. Untreated strabismus and hypermetropia can be associated with amblyopia. All cases of suspected strabismus need orthoptic and ophthalmic assessment.

13.2 Divergent Strabismus (Exotropia)

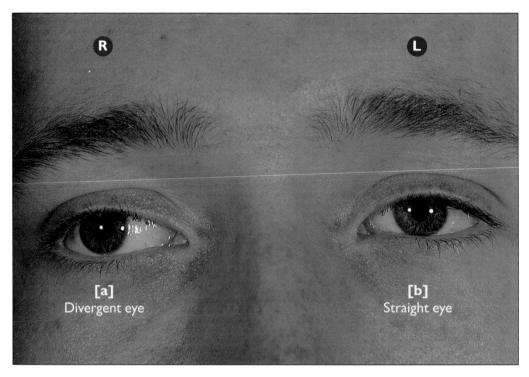

R   L

[a]
Divergent eye

[b]
Straight eye

Right divergent strabismus (exotropia)

Divergent strabismus (DS) in children is much less common than convergent strabismus (see 13.1). A small percentage of children with divergent strabismus may have **serious ophthalmic or neurological** disease manifesting as strabismus, and the examiner should be alert to this possibility. Divergent strabismus may also present in young adults (especially myopes). Symptoms may be intermittent and precipitated by periods of intensive study. In older patients, divergent strabismus may occur in any eye that has long-term loss of vision.

13.3 Vertical Strabismus (Hypertropia)

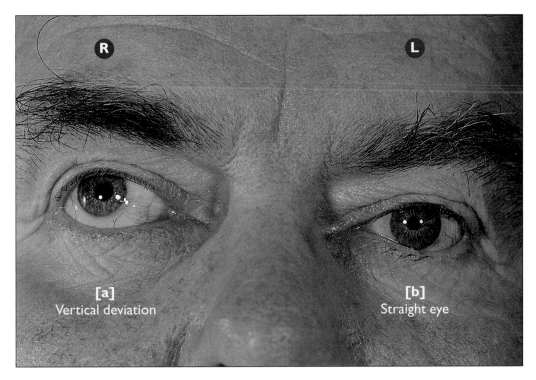

R

L

[a]
Vertical deviation

[b]
Straight eye

Right vertical strabismus (hypertropia)

Although vertical strabismus is not common, it is usually associated with **significant orbital disease** such as thyroid eye disease (see 6.13), inflammation, tumours and fractures of the orbital floor (see 6.15). Patients need a careful systemic work up.

13.4 Amblyopia – Occlusion Therapy

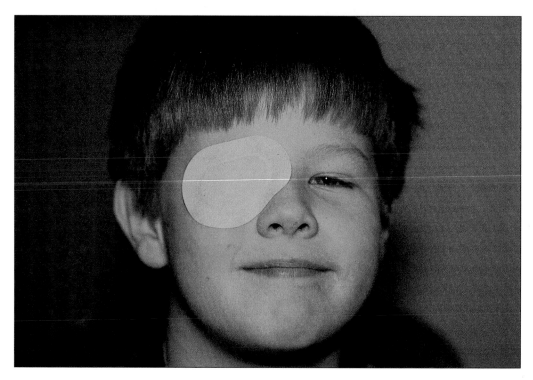

Total occlusion with a patch

Amblyopia (**'lazy eye'**) is a deficit of formed vision in an anatomically normal eye. Causes include uncorrected refractive errors, myopia and hypermetropia (see 5.1 and 5.2), strabismus (see 13.1 and 13.2) and media opacity. Children under the age of 7 years (the sensitive period) are at risk of amblyopia as the visual system is still developing. Therapy aims to make the child use the lazy eye by **occluding** the good eye, and correcting any refractive errors. Early identification and therapy are vital if this condition is to be successfully treated. Once the sensitive period has passed, treatment will not be useful.

13.5 Prism Cover Test

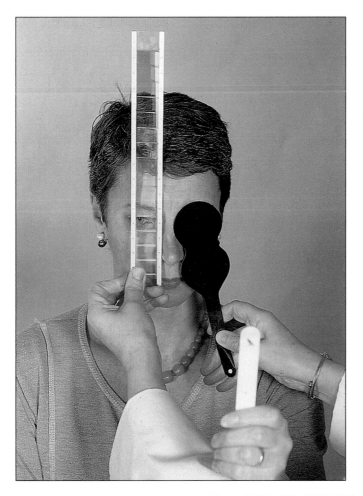

Patient fixes on a target while the examiner corrects the strabismus with a prism

It is extremely helpful to be able to **quantify** the **angle** of an ocular deviation, particularly if surgical intervention is planned. The size of a deviation can be measured in either degrees or prism dioptres, and the technique most commonly used is the **prism cover test** (PCT). During a PCT an alternate cover test is performed whilst prisms of increasing power are placed before one eye, until the ocular deviation is neutralised. Serial PCTs can demonstrate whether the angle of an ocular deviation is stable or changing, for example, in thyroid eye disease.

13.6 Synoptophore

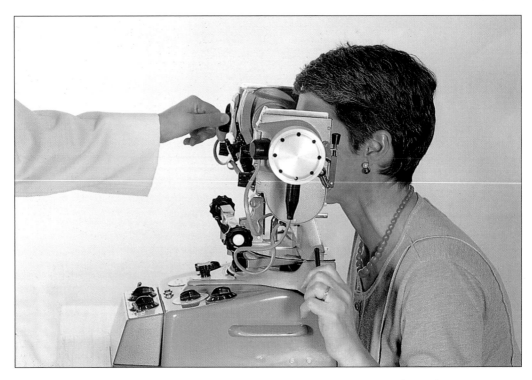

Patient looks at images in the synoptophore allowing the examiner to assess the strabismus

The **synoptophore** is an instrument used by **orthoptists** when assessing **strabismus** and **binocular function**. One can measure the **angle of deviation** of the eyes, check the ability of the eyes to **fuse** disparate images, detect **suppression** of images (in amblyopia) and assess the degree of **stereopsis** present in patients with strabismus. The instrument essentially consists of two hollow tubes containing mirrors and children often enjoy 'playing' on the machine. The subject is asked to perform tasks such as 'putting a lion in a cage'.

14.1 Ophthalmia Neonatorum (Conjunctivitis of the Newborn)

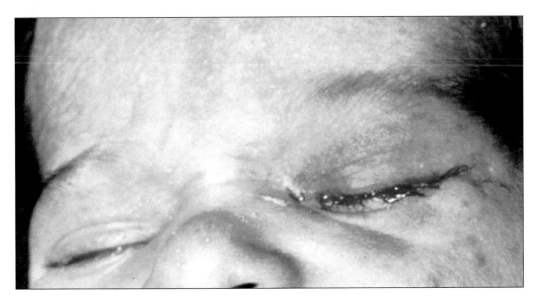

Purulent conjunctivitis in the first week requires urgent referral and is notifiable

Purulent conjunctivitis occurs in about 2% of neonates in developed countries. The period of time between birth and presentation is variable in the first two weeks. Pathogens include **Gonococci**, **Chlamydia trachomatis**, Haemophilus species, Staphylococcus aureus and Streptococcus pneumoniae. **Congenital nasolacrimal obstruction** is also associated with neonatal conjunctivitis. Some of the pathogens listed above can cause **severe** disease, and may lead to corneal infection or marked **systemic disease**. For this reason, all neonates with a purulent conjunctivitis need careful assessment and follow up. Ophthalmia neonatorum is a **notifiable disease**. It is important to exclude infection in both parents.

14.2 Leukocoria – Retinoblastoma

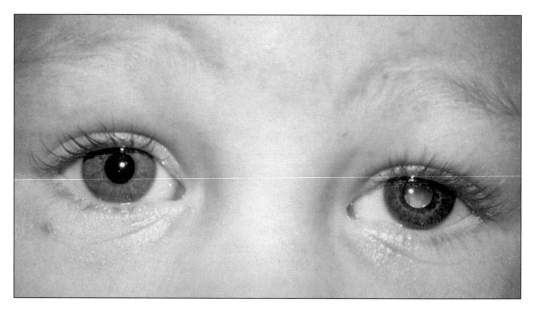

White pupil on the left side – retinoblastoma

The term **leukocoria** refers to the clinical sign of a **white pupil** with **no red reflex**, and is usually detected in a newborn or young child. Leukocoria is an extremely serious sign as it may signify the presence of **life-threatening** pathology. **Retinoblastoma** is a malignant **intraocular tumour** of primitive retinal cells (with unilateral and bilateral forms) which invades the central nervous system via the optic nerve, and is usually fatal without treatment. Any child with leukocoria needs **urgent** assessment. Some cases are detected because white reflexes are noticed on flash photography, although most white reflexes detected this way are due to light reflected off the optic disc.

Differential Diagnosis of Leukocoria	
Congenital cataract	14.3
Retinoblastoma	
Retinopathy of prematurity	14.4
Toxocara infection	
Coloboma	2.2
Persistent hyperplastic primary vitreous	

14.3 Congenital Cataract

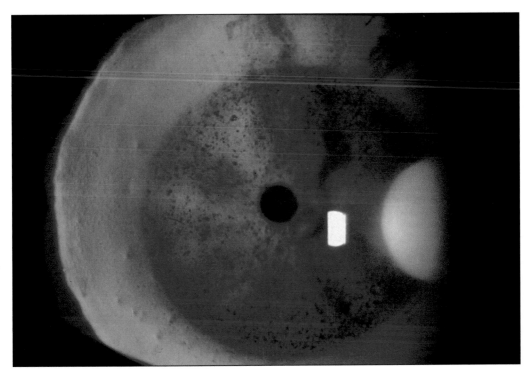

Dark area on the red reflex is a congenital cataract

Congenital cataract may be idiopathic, inherited, associated with intrauterine infections or metabolic disorders, or may occur as part of ocular, systemic or other chromosomal disease. Dense cataract will cause leukocoria. Cataract may be unilateral or bilateral and lead to reduced visual input and associated amblyopia. Successful management of patients with lens opacity is dependent on early detection and urgent referral of affected children.

Causes of Infantile Cataract

Idiopathic
Infection during pregnancy (e.g. rubella)
Metabolic (e.g. galactosaemia)
Associated with other ocular disease (e.g. microphthalmos, ROP)
Inherited   a) isolated cataract
            b) with systemic disease (e.g. Trisomy 21)
Drug induced (e.g. steroids)
Trauma

14.4 Retinopathy of Prematurity

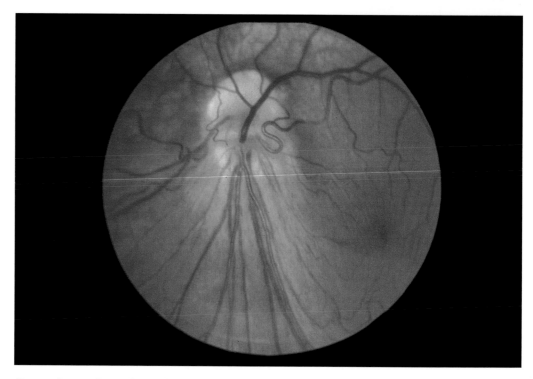

'Dragged' optic disc and macula due to peripheral scarring and contraction of the retina

Retinopathy of prematurity (ROP) is a disease of the immature retina and retinal vasculature associated with **prematurity** and **low birth weight**. Abnormal retinal vessels proliferate in ROP and lead to haemorrhage, cicatricial changes and **retinal detachment**. ROP was initially thought to be caused by the oxygen used in special care units, but it is now apparent that the pathogenesis of the disease is more complex than this. All babies at risk of developing ROP are now **screened** by ophthalmic surgeons according to defined protocols.

14.5 Retinopathy of Prematurity – Treatment

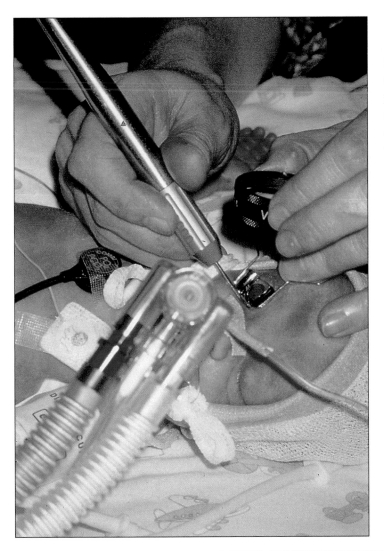

Cryotherapy for treatment of retinopathy of prematurity being performed in intensive care while the baby continues to be ventilated

There are strict criteria for the treatment of ROP. Once the clinical disease has progressed to a **threshold** stage, as determined by fundal examination, then the benefits of intervention outweigh the risks of treatment. In order to arrest disease progression it is necessary to **ablate** the **peripheral ischaemic retina** with either **laser** or **cryotherapy**. Treatment is technically difficult and is often performed on infants who are extremely unwell.

14.6 Infantile Glaucoma – Buphthalmos

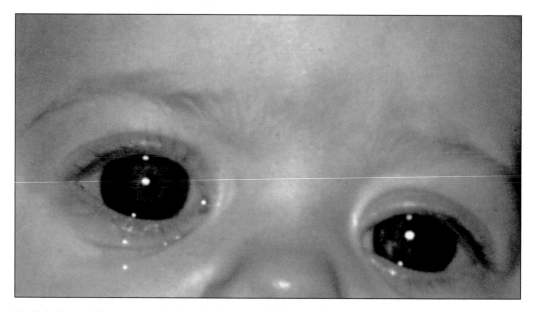

Buphthalmos with tearing and photophobia in a child. Note the asymmetrically enlarged eyes

Children with **infantile glaucoma** usually present in the **first year** of life, and features include large **(buphthalmic)** eye(s), **watery** eye(s), **corneal clouding**, **photophobia** and blepharospasm. Glaucoma in infants is extremely **rare** and many of the symptoms, such as watery eyes, occur in conditions which are seen commonly such as **nasolacrimal obstruction**. However, the consequences of missing a diagnosis of infantile glaucoma may have serious implications for visual potential, and it is extremely important to consider infantile glaucoma in the **differential diagnosis** of children presenting with large or watery eyes. Disease may be bilateral, but with marked asymmetry between the two eyes.

14.7 Microphthalmos

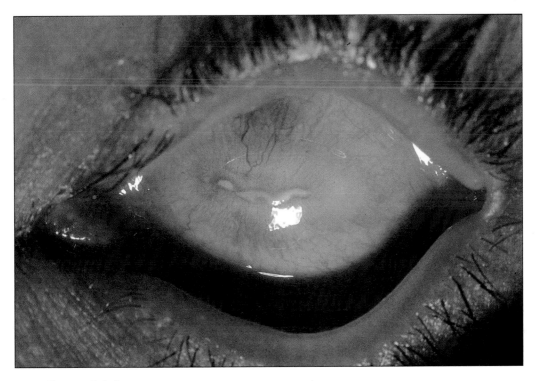

A small microphthalmic eye

In **microphthalmos** one or both eyes are abnormally small due to problems during ocular development *in utero*. Microphthalmic eyes may also have uveal **colobomas**. Patients may have **chromosomal** or other **systemic abnormalities**, including cardiac defects. The correction of **refractive errors** and management of **amblyopia** are important if appropriate.

14.8 Congenital Dystrophic Ptosis

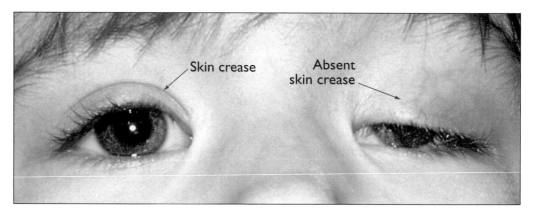

Skin crease

Absent skin crease

Drooping of left upper eyelid covering pupil can cause amblyopia

Congenital dystrophic ptosis is caused by a **developmental anomaly** of the levator palpebrae superioris muscle/tendon complex. There may be an associated **astigmatic refractive error** (see 5.4) and children may develop **amblyopia** (see 13.4). The management of ptosis depends on the degree of ptosis and the amount of residual muscle function. Most ophthalmologists plan surgical correction between the ages of 2 and 4. Earlier surgery is needed if the upper lid is covering the visual axis.

15.1 Normal Optic Disc and Optic Atrophy

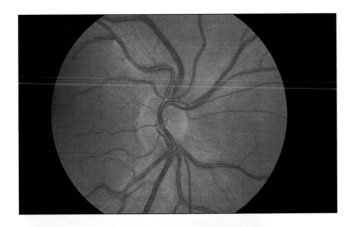

Normal optic disc

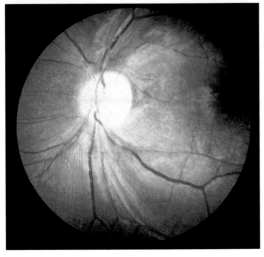

Optic atrophy – pale white disc

A normal optic disc should be pink with a clearly defined edge. In **optic atrophy** the most striking feature is the **pallor** of the disc.

> Causes of Optic Atrophy
>
> Glaucoma (optic atrophy and cupping)
> Ischaemia
> Drug Toxicity
> Demyelination
> Trauma
> Compression of the anterior visual pathway – tumour
>   – aneurysm
> Viral infections
> Retinal dystrophy (e.g. RP)
> Hereditary forms

15.2 Normal Optic Disc and Swollen Optic Disc

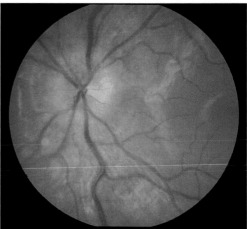

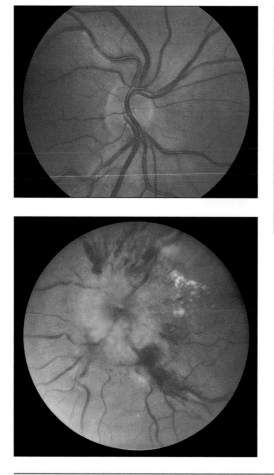

(top left) Normal optic disc

(above) Swelling of the optic disc with blurred disc margin and loss of optic cup

(left) Advanced swelling of the optic disc with flame haemorrhages, yellow exudates and white swollen retina

When the optic disc is swollen the margin of the disc is indistinct and the disc may appear elevated. The central cup region of the disc may be obliterated by swollen tissue, and the retinal venules may be dilated, tortuous and pulsation is absent. One should determine whether the disc swelling is unilateral or bilateral. The differential diagnosis of a swollen disc includes papilloedema, central retinal venous occlusion, optic neuritis, hypertension, ischaemic optic neuropathy (see 15.3), infiltration of the nerve, for example, sarcoid, tumours of the nerve and orbital compression, for example, thyroid eye disease. Visual acuity is characteristically, but not invariably, preserved in papilloedema despite marked optic disc swelling.

15.3 Normal Optic Disc and Anterior Ischaemic Optic Neuropathy

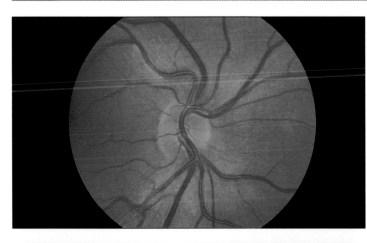

Normal optic disc

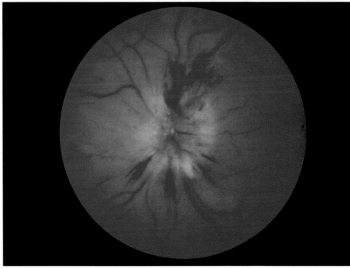

Swollen and pale optic disc with surrounding haemorrhages in temporal arteritis

Anterior ischaemic optic neuropathy (AION) results from occlusion of the blood supply to the optic nerve head. Patients present with **sudden loss of vision** in the affected eye, and the optic disc is usually **pale and swollen**. Peri-disc splinter haemorrhages are often seen. About 10% of patients with AION will have **giant cell arteritis** (see 15.14), and it is essential to exclude this **blinding** disease. The other 90% of patients with non-arteritic AION may have **systemic** conditions such as **hypertension**, diabetes, hyperlipidaemia or hyperviscosity.

15.4 Bitemporal Hemianopia due to Chiasmal Compression

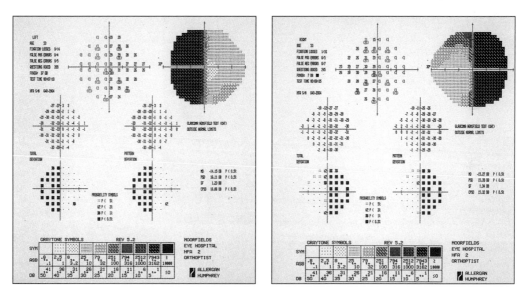

Computerised perimetry showing a bitemporal hemianopia due to pituitary adenoma

Bitemporal hemianopia is the classical visual field defect seen in patients with lesions or compression of the **optic chiasm**. The defect is produced because of the anatomical **decussation** of fibres at the chiasm (see 3.4). Lesions which may compress the chiasm include **pituitary tumours**, aneurysms, optic nerve and chiasmal gliomas, craniopharyngiomas and distension of the third ventricle in obstructive hydrocephalus. Visual field defects can be identified quickly with a simple **confrontation test** using a red target (see 4.10). Patients with bitemporal hemianopias are not eligible to drive.

15.5 Homonymous Quadrantanopia

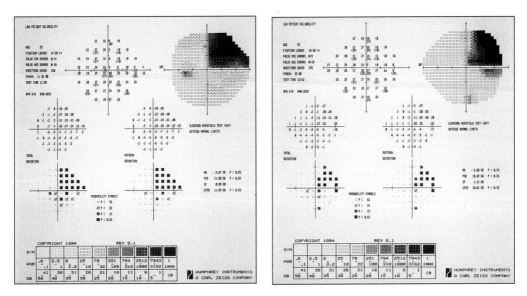

Computerised perimetry – homonymous quadrantanopia due to a stroke

Homonymous quadrantanopias are caused by **retro-chiasmal** lesions of the visual pathway (see 3.4). Common causes include **cerebrovascular events** and space-occupying lesions. It is important to test the visual fields to confrontation in all cases of **unexplained visual loss**, since patients are often not fully aware of their field defect. In lesions of the visual (occipital) cortex there may be preservation of visual acuity if there is 'macular sparing'. The visual field defect may be a quadrantanopia or a hemianopia depending on the extent and exact position of the intracranial pathology. Patients with homonymous quadrantanopias (encroaching close to the midline) are not eligible to drive.

15.6 Third Cranial Nerve Palsy

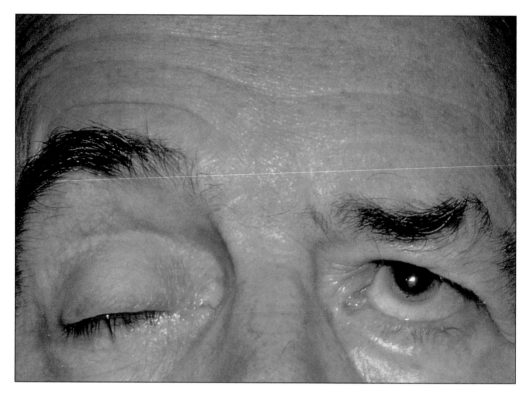

Right third cranial nerve palsy with complete ptosis caused by intracranial aneurysm

The signs of a **third cranial nerve** (CNIII) **palsy** include **ptosis, pupil dilation**, and **exotropic** and **hypotropic** (depressed) globe position ('down and out'). **Congenital** CNIII palsies do not involve the pupil. **Acquired** causes include brainstem lesions, inflammation, vascular lesions (a **painful** CNIII palsy with involvement of the **pupil** suggests an intracranial **aneurysm**), tumours, **diabetes** (usually no pupil involvement) and **major trauma**.

15.7 Fourth Cranial Nerve Palsy

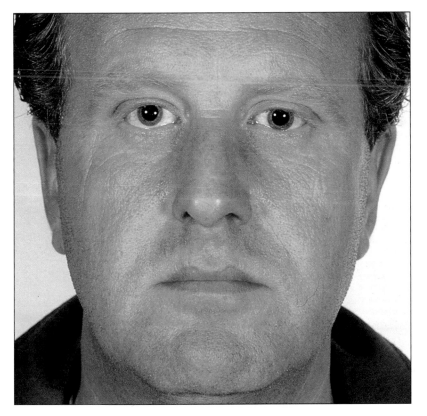

Fourth cranial nerve palsy – right hypertropia (see inferior scleral show) due to trauma

Fourth cranial nerve palsies can be difficult to diagnose. In acute lesions, patients often complain of a combination of vertical, horizontal and torsional **diplopia**. Symptoms may be worse on looking downwards, for example, when going down stairs or reading. Signs may be subtle and include a compensatory **head posture** to overcome diplopia (head tilt and face turn to opposite side and chin depression). Cover testing reveals an **ipsilateral hypertropia**. The patient shown has a small vertical ocular deviation, with the right eye higher than the left (Right IVth nerve palsy). Causes include **congenital lesions** (30%), **head trauma** (30%), ischaemia (20%) and intracranial neoplasia and aneurysms (5%). Bilateral fourth nerve palsies (often after trauma) are difficult to diagnose as they are usually only manifest when patients perform activities such as reading, and are easily missed if a careful history is not taken.

15.8 Sixth Cranial Nerve Palsy

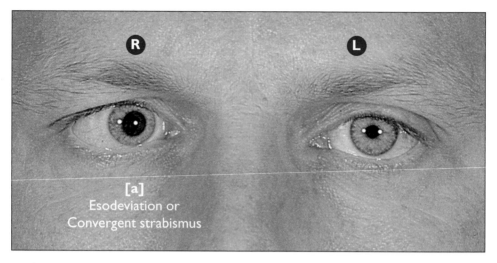

Sixth cranial nerve palsy – right esotropia in the primary position (patient looking straight ahead)

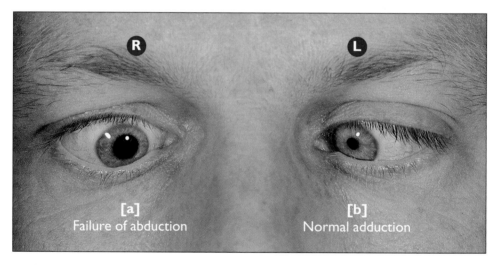

Sixth cranial nerve palsy – failure of attempted right eye abduction when patient asked to look to the right

Patients with an acquired sixth cranial nerve palsy present with **horizontal diplopia**, an ipsilateral **esotropia** in the primary position and **limitation of abduction** of the affected eye. Causes include **ischaemia**, aneurysms, diabetes mellitus, demyelination, middle ear infections and intracranial inflammatory diseases.

15.9 Seventh Cranial Nerve Palsy

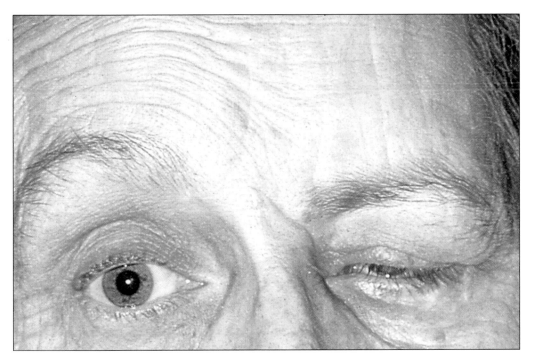

Seventh cranial nerve palsy – inability to use left frontalis muscle (lower motor neurone)

Seventh cranial nerve palsy may be due to **upper** (forehead frontalis muscle spared) or **lower motor neurone** lesions. Signs include incomplete eyelid closure **(lagophthalmos)**, lower lid paralytic ectropion, epiphora, **nocturnal** lagophthalmos and **corneal exposure**. It is extremely important to identify and treat the patient at risk of corneal exposure and **ulceration**

15.10 Heterochromia Iridis

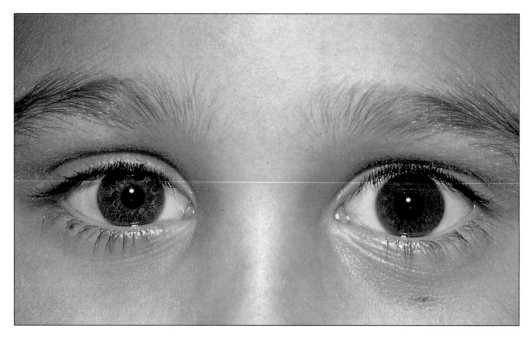

Abnormal iris is pale due to congenital Horner's syndrome

A difference in colour between the two irides **(heterochromia iridis)** may be congenital or acquired. **Congenital causes** include an idiopathic form and congenital Horner's syndrome (shown above). **Acquired causes** include Fuch's heterochromic cyclitis (an idiopathic unilateral inflammatory condition), Herpes zoster infection (see 6.12), trauma, siderosis from a retained iron metallic intraocular foreign body, with the use of prostaglandin analogue glaucoma eye drops, and iris melanoma (see 12.4).

15.11 Anisocoria

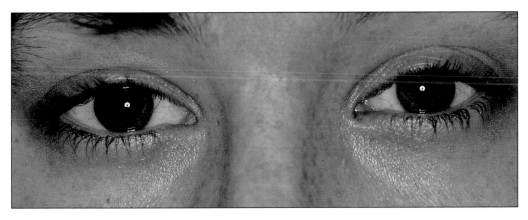

Different sized pupils – neurological examination is required to determine the abnormal eye and cause

Anisocoria refers to a difference in the size of the pupils. **Simple** anisocoria (difference should be less than 1 mm) occurs in about 25% of the population, and apart from the unequal size the pupils are otherwise normal. **Acquired** causes of anisocoria (difference usually greater than 1 mm) include eye drops, Horner's syndrome (see 15.12), third cranial nerve palsy (see 15.6) and Holmes–Adie syndrome.

15.12 Horner's Syndrome

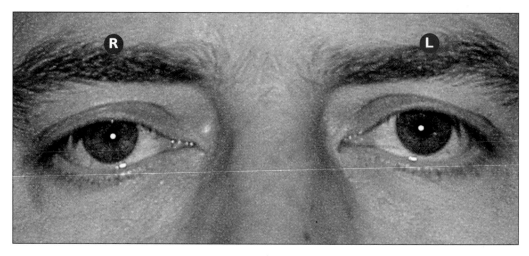

Right eye has drooping upper lid and small pupil. Full neurological examination is required to determine the cause

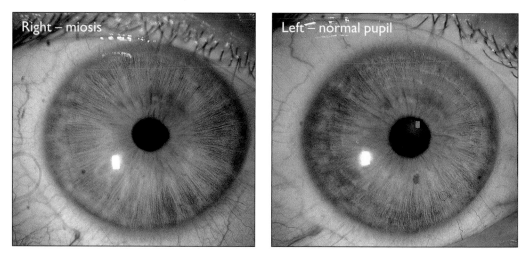

Right – miosis

Left – normal pupil

Pupil asymmetry in Horner's syndrome

Horner's syndrome is caused by an interruption to the sympathetic innervation to the eye at any point between the hypothalamus and the orbit. Clinical signs include slight ptosis (1 to 2 mm), pupil miosis and reduced sweating of the ipsilateral face and neck. If the lesion is congenital or occurs during early infancy then heterochromia iridis (see 15.10) may be present. There are a range of possible causes including cerebrovascular events, neoplasia, demyelination, infection and inflammation, which can occur at any point along the pathway.

15.13 Myasthenia Gravis

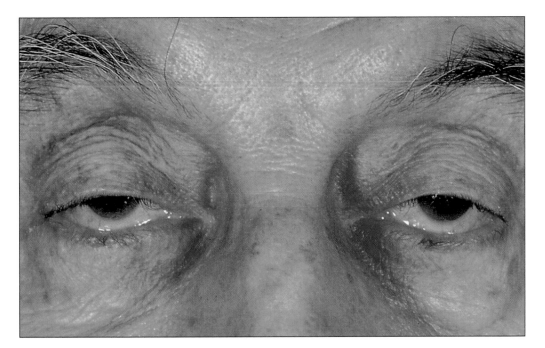

Bilateral (variable) ptosis in myasthenia gravis

Myasthenia gravis is a rare systemic condition characterised by a progressive inability to sustain contractions of skeletal muscle. Patients often present with signs of ophthalmic involvement, and may have **variable ptosis** and **diplopia**. Ptosis is usually **bilateral**. Systemic features include proximal muscle weakness, difficulty in swallowing and dysarthria. Symptoms are worse at the end of the day from fatigue. **Autoantibodies** against the acetylcholine receptor are present in over 95% of cases. Some patients have a rapid deterioration in their condition **(myasthenic crisis)** and need **urgent (same day)** hospital admission.

15.14 Giant Cell Arteritis

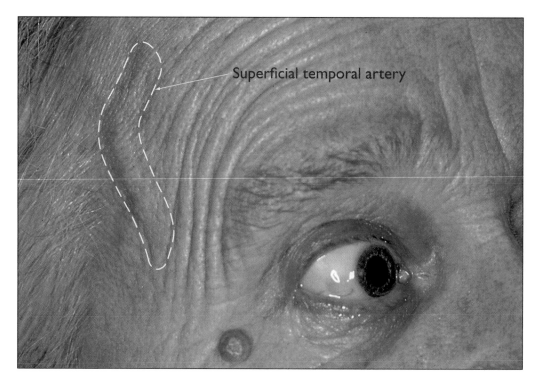

Superficial temporal artery

Enlarged tender superficial temporal artery in giant cell arteritis

Giant cell arteritis is a necrotising systemic **vasculitis** with a predilection for the cranial arteries. Patients are often unwell with fatigue, weight loss and severe focal **hemicranial headache**, often localised over branches of the superficial temporal artery – which may be enlarged, tender and nodular with reduced pulsation. **Claudication** of the **jaw** and **tongue** are pathognomonic. Patients may have symptoms of polymyalgia rheumatica (including pain in proximal muscles, the shoulder girdle and hip). **Visual loss**, due to **anterior ischaemic optic neuropathy**, is usually sudden and severe. Unless **immediate** high dose **corticosteroid** therapy is started, **irreversible, bilateral** visual loss may occur. **Urgent (same day)** referral for admission, temporal artery biopsy and management is needed.

16.1 Operating Microscope

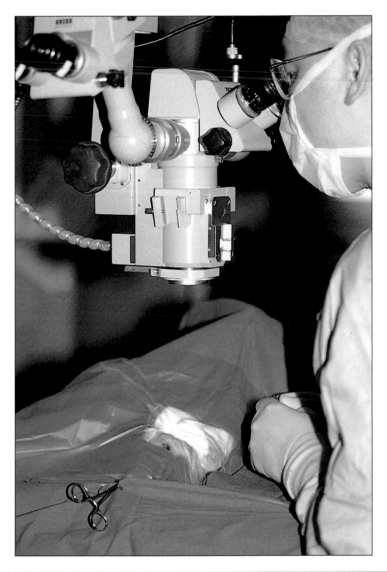

Binocular operating microscope in position at start of surgery

The development of the binocular **operating microscope** (OM) has revolutionised ophthalmic surgery. All **intraocular surgery** is now performed under the OM with high levels of precision and safety. The magnification produced by the OM allows surgeons to operate with controlled movements down to the order of 200 micrometres.

16.2 Microsurgical Instrumentation

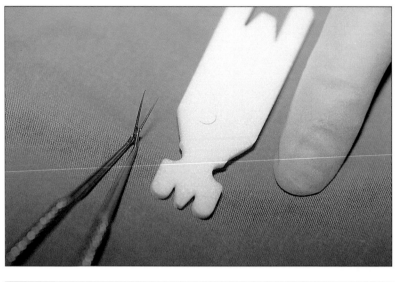

Capsule forceps and 10/0 nylon microsurgical suture used in cataract surgery

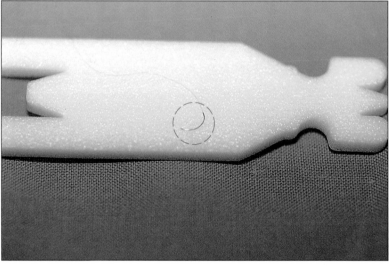

10/0 nylon microsurgical suture used for suturing cornea and sclera

Modern microsurgical instruments enable the surgeon to operate within the eye with a high degree of precision. The capsulorhexis forceps shown enable the surgeon to create a circular tear in the anterior capsule of the lens, in order to gain access to the nuclear material of the lens in phacoemulsification cataract surgery (see 16.6).

The suture material in routine use for corneal stitches after cataract surgery is a **10/0 Nylon monofilament** suture, which is just visible to the naked eye. Nylon sutures have high tensile strength and degrade slowly. Loose or broken sutures are a common cause of foreign body sensations in patients who have had previous intraocular surgery.

16.3 Local Anaesthesia – Peribulbar Injection

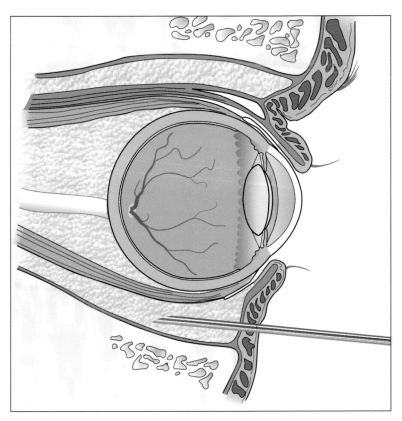

Pre-operative injection through lower lid to anaesthetise eye

About 75% of all ophthalmic surgery is performed as a day case under **local anaesthesia**. One of the commonest local anaesthetic (LA) techniques used is **peribulbar injection**. This method involves inserting a needle approximately 2 cm into the orbit to the region of the **equator** of the globe. After injection of about 5 mls of LA a small **compression** weight is placed on the eye to facilitate diffusion of the solution around the globe. There is a small risk of **perforation** of the globe during all LA **injection** techniques. Alternative local anaesthetic techniques include operating under topical anaesthesia, or using retrobulbar or sub–Tenon's anaesthesia.

16.4 Intraocular Lenses

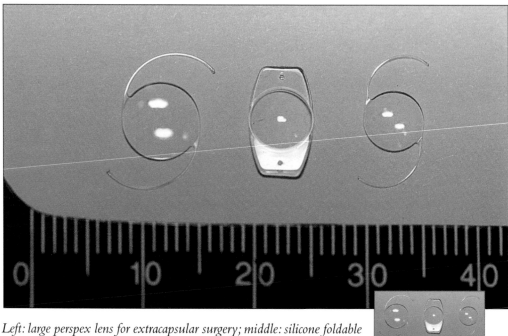

Left: large perspex lens for extracapsular surgery; middle: silicone foldable lens and right: small perspex lens, both for phacoemulsification

Actual Size

The development of implantable **intraocular lenses** (IOLs) has revolutionised **cataract surgery** in the latter half of this century. Rigid lenses made from inert Polymethylmethacrylate (perspex) are used in extracapsular cataract surgery. With the advent of ultrasonic fragmentation of cataracts **(phacoemulsification)** in small incision surgery, there has been the development of **foldable and injectable IOLs** made from **silicone** and **acrylic**-based materials, which can be inserted into the capsular bag through very small incisions (3.5 mm or less).

16.5 Cataract Surgery – Extracapsular Approach with Post-Operative Iris Prolapse

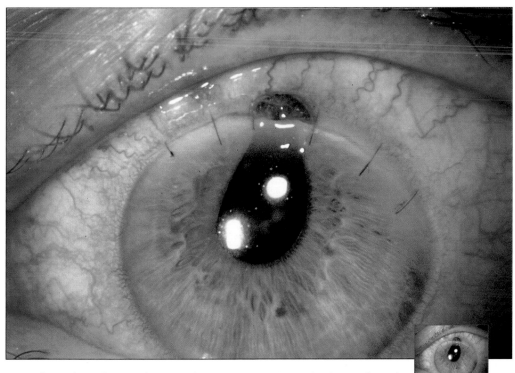

Iris prolapse through corneal incision between sutures. Note the distorted pupil　　*Actual size*

In extracapsular cataract surgery the incision into the eye is up to 11 mm long and is usually sutured with five 10/0 Nylon sutures. Blunt trauma to the eye in the post-operative period can lead to **wound dehiscence** and an **iris prolapse** (note the peaked pupil in the illustration above). **Urgent (same day) surgical intervention** is necessary to repair the wound.

16.6 Cataract Surgery – Phacoemulsification

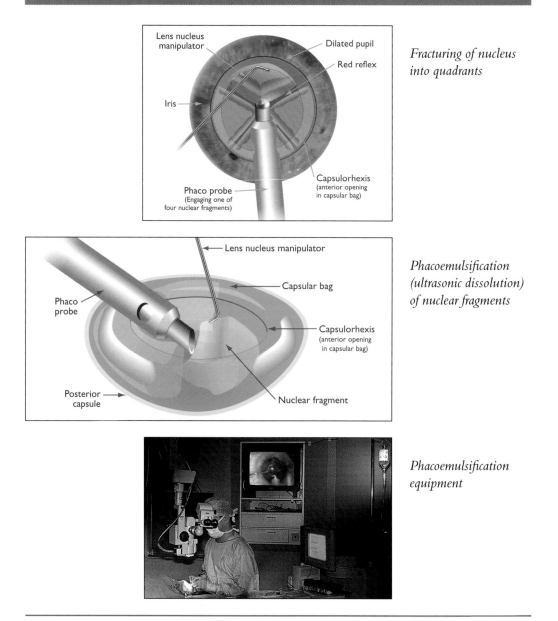

Lens nucleus manipulator

Dilated pupil

Red reflex

Iris

Capsulorhexis
(anterior opening in capsular bag)

Phaco probe
(Engaging one of four nuclear fragments)

Fracturing of nucleus into quadrants

Lens nucleus manipulator

Capsular bag

Phaco probe

Capsulorhexis
(anterior opening in capsular bag)

Posterior capsule

Nuclear fragment

Phacoemulsification (ultrasonic dissolution) of nuclear fragments

Phacoemulsification equipment

The advent of small incision, sutureless cataract surgery enables the removal of a cataract and insertion of an intraocular lens (IOL) to be performed through an incision of approximately 3 mm width. The cataract is fragmented with an ultrasonic probe within the capsular bag, and an IOL (see 16.4) can then be placed within the normal lens capsular bag. Visual rehabilitation is usually rapid, with low levels of post-operative astigmatism (see 5.4)

16.7 Cataract Surgery – Post-operative YAG Laser Posterior Capsulotomy

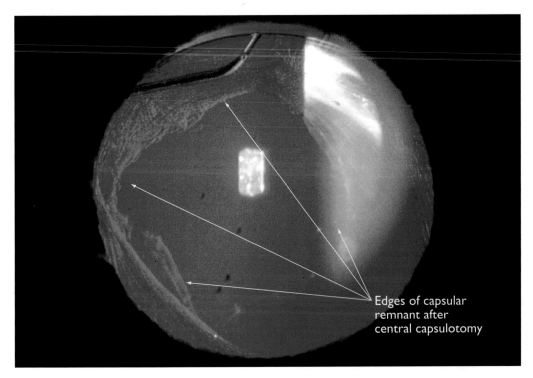

Edges of capsular remnant after central capsulotomy

The opaque posterior capsule has been cut away with a laser to clear the visual axis

Implantation of the intraocular lens within the capsular bag provides a high degree of lens **stability**. In about **20%** of patients the posterior capsule can progressively opacify due to proliferation of remaining lens cells, usually within 12 to 18 months of surgery. Patients report that their vision has decreased from the immediate post-operative result. It is possible to perform a YAG laser capsulotomy as an out-patient procedure and remove the scar tissue from the visual axis. There is a small incidence (approximately 1%) of **retinal detachment** (see 11.1) after this procedure.

16.8 Glaucoma Filtration Surgery – Trabeculectomy

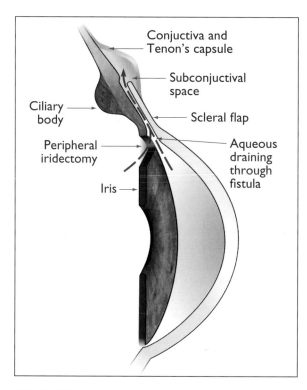

Conjuctiva and
Tenon's capsule

Subconjuctival
space

Ciliary
body

Scleral flap

Peripheral
iridectomy

Aqueous
draining
through
fistula

Iris

Creation of drainage channel

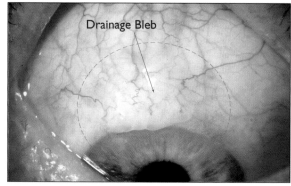

Drainage Bleb

Post-operative appearance of 'bleb' – conjunctiva with aqueous under it

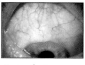

Actual size

Trabeculectomy is the **standard glaucoma filtration procedure**, which creates a 'trap-door' valve in the sclera between the anterior chamber and the subconjunctival space, diverting aqueous and reducing the intraocular pressure. **Post-operative scarring** may prevent aqueous flow, and a variety of adjuvant therapies can be used to reduce scarring, including the single, intra-operative application of anti-cancer agents on a sponge: **5-Fluorouracil** (5-FU) **and Mitomycin C** (MMC) and the post-operative injection of 5-FU under the conjunctiva. The use of these agents necessitates more frequent observation in the early post-operative period.

16.9 Trabeculectomy – Post-operative Bleb Infection and Endophthalmitis

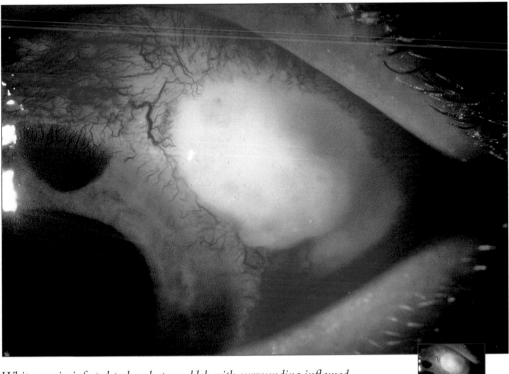

White pus in infected trabeculectomy bleb with surrounding inflamed conjunctiva

Actual size

Adjuvant **antimetabolite therapy**, for example, 5-FU or MMC, may be used in patients who have a high risk of their trabeculectomy failing from post-operative subconjunctival scarring. Some patients develop a **thin, cystic drainage bleb** after surgery, particularly if antimetabolites have been used. These eyes are at **life-long risk** of developing **bleb infections** and **endophthalmitis**, and any **purulent discharge** or pain from the eye that has had previous filtration surgery needs to be managed with **intensive topical antibiotics** and **immediate (same day)** ophthalmic referral.

16.10 Corneal Transplantation (Penetrating Keratoplasty)

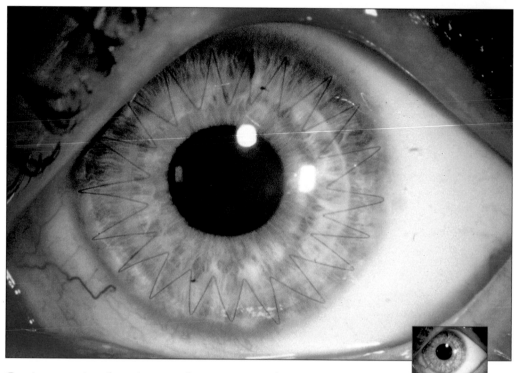

Continuous 10/0 nylon microsurgical suture in corneal transplant

Actual size

Corneal transplantation is an effective technique for replacing a cornea that has severe irreversible opacification or damage. Corneal graft survival and visual rehabilitation are particularly good in patients with **corneal dystrophies** such as keratoconus and Fuch's endothelial dystrophies. Visual rehabilitation may take several months after surgery, and **suture adjustment** may be needed to control graft **astigmatism** (see 5.4). Corneal **graft rejection** (see 16.11) can occur at any time after a penetrating keratoplasty.

16.11 Acute Corneal Graft Rejection

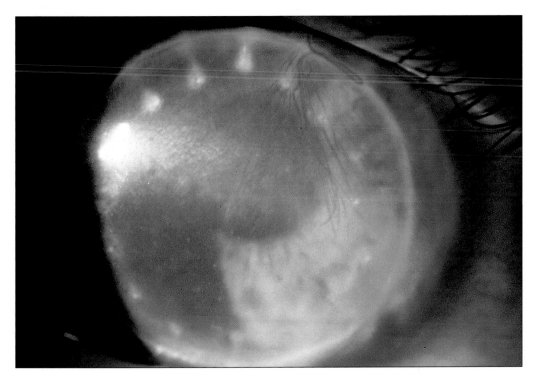

Corneal graft rejection in a vascularised graft

All patients who have had a penetrating keratoplasty are at **life-long risk** of graft rejection. **Loose or broken sutures** are a frequent cause of rejection episodes. Any conjunctival injection, gritty pain or reduced vision in a grafted eye should be managed as a possible rejection episode, with **immediate** ophthalmic referral. **Intensive** treatment with **topical steroid therapy** can reverse most rejection episodes.

16.12 Refractive Surgery – Lasik

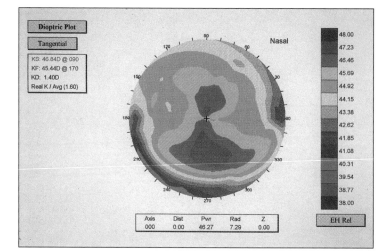

a) Corneal topographic map – computer picture of the shape of the corneal surface

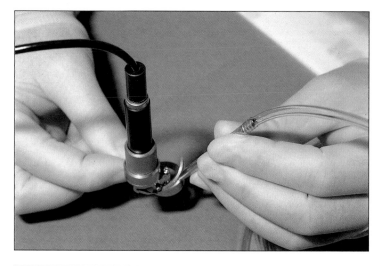

b) Microkeratome – precision blade to cut a flap in the cornea

Lasik (laser in-situ keratomileusis) is a recent **refractive** surgical technique in which an area of central cornea is ablated with a laser, which alters the shape and refractive power of the cornea and therefore the refractive status of the eye. An extremely precise **microkeratome** (b) is used to cut a very thin slice of central cornea (c) that is hinged at one side (d). The corneal flap is laid to one side and the underlying corneal stroma is lasered (e). The **corneal flap** is then replaced. Lasik has the advantages of less post-operative corneal haze and scarring, more rapid visual rehabilitation, and the corneal epithelium is not removed during treatment.

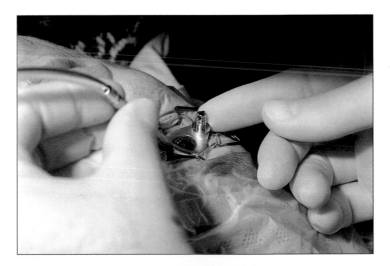

c) The microkeratome is put on the eye and a flap is cut in the cornea

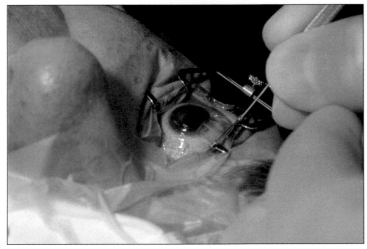

d) The flap of cornea is held back, hinged at its upper edge

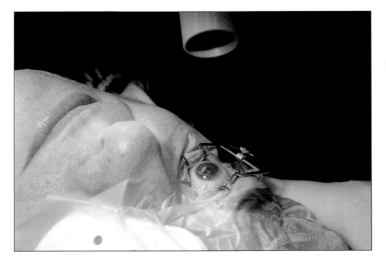

e) The cornea under the flap is remodelled with the laser

16.13 Refractive Surgery – Photo-refractive Keratectomy

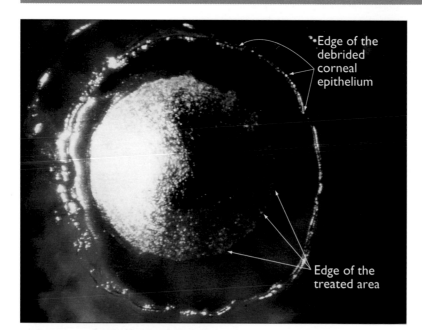

• Edge of the debrided corneal epithelium

Edge of the treated area

The corneal epithelium has been removed and the laser has remodelled a precise area of the corneal stroma

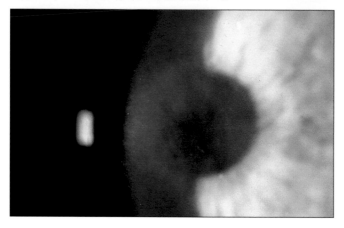

A grey scar has formed in the corneal area treated by the laser

Photo-refractive keratectomy (PRK) is a refractive surgical procedure in which a laser is used to ablate and remodel an area of **central cornea**. By altering corneal shape one can change the refractive power of the cornea and correct refractive errors. PRK provides predictable results for low to moderate degrees of myopia, but is less predictable in high refractive errors. It is necessary to remove the corneal epithelium in PRK, which can cause marked post-operative pain. All refractive procedures carry the risk of **complications** including severe infections. Corneal stromal haze and scarring may occur after PRK as shown in the illustration.

16.14 Refractive Surgery – Radial Keratotomy

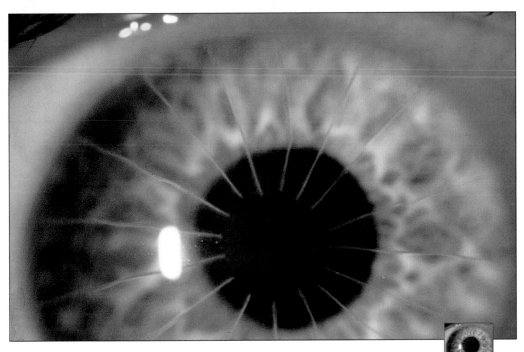

The cornea is flattened by multiple radial incisions reducing the myopia

Actual size

Radial keratotomy is a refractive surgical technique used to correct myopia (see 5.1). The principle of the operation is to induce **flattening** of the **cornea** by means of deep partial thickness **radial incisions** in the corneal stroma. This technique is not suitable for correcting high myopia (greater than 8 dioptres). **Complications** include a reduction in best corrected visual acuity (in about 10% of patients), glare, occasional unpredictable refractive outcome, reduction in the mechanical strength of the cornea and risk of serious corneal infection.

16.15 Strabismus Surgery – Horizontal Recess/Resect Procedures

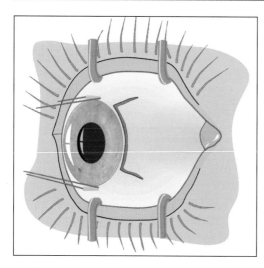

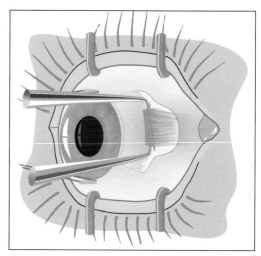

Red line indicates incision in conjunctiva over medial rectus muscle

The medial rectus is held on a squint hook

The cut muscle is reattached further back on the eye to effectively weaken it

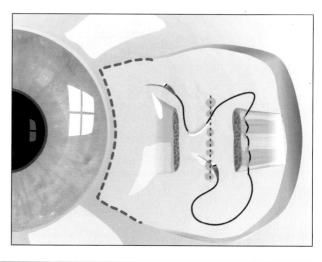

Most forms of **horizontal** strabismus surgery for **convergent** or **divergent** squints involve operating on the medial/lateral rectus muscles. Muscles are either weakened by **recession** (set back) from their original insertion or strengthened by **resection** (shortened) and reattached to their original insertion. The amount of surgery performed is based on the **measured angle** of the strabismus (see 13.5). More than one procedure may be required for very large squints. In difficult cases, for example, thyroid eye disease (see 6.13), the sutures are tied so that one can **adjust** the eye position with the patient awake.

16.16 Retinal Detachment Surgery – Cryotherapy and Scleral Explant

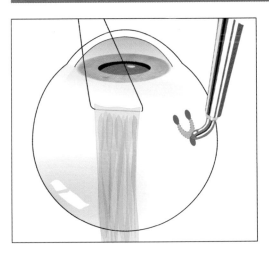

Cryotherapy (freezing treatment) is applied to the sclera

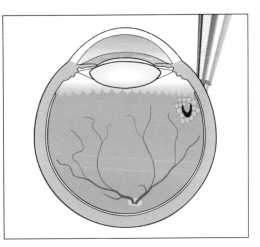

The cryotherapy causes scarring which seals the retinal hole

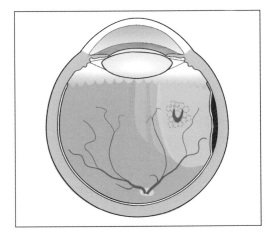

Cryotherapy is used to treat the retinal hole causing the retinal detachment

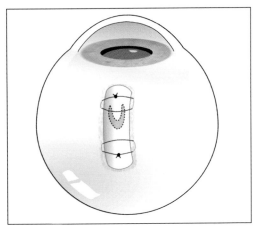

A piece of silicone is stitched to the sclera to close the retinal hole

One of the principles of retinal detachment surgery is that any retinal breaks (see 11.1) must be closed. Closure of the retinal tear can often be achieved by means of external indentation of the globe by an explant sutured to the sclera. When combined with retinal cryotherapy to seal the closed tear, this is a very effective technique for many primary forms of retinal detachment. Surgery may also involve drainage of subretinal fluid and injection of intraocular air or expansile gas. Patients who have had intraocular gas will be advised by their surgeon about the period of time (several weeks) for which they cannot fly in aircraft.

16.17 Retinal Detachment Surgery – Vitrectomy

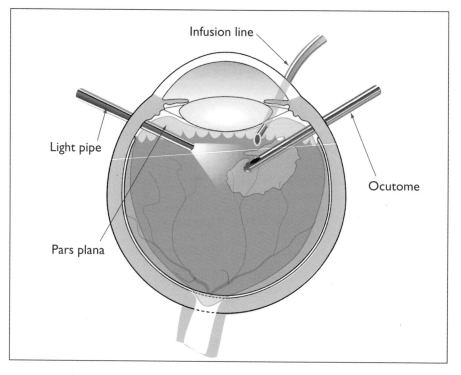

Microsurgical instruments cut the vitreous gel from the eye

Pars plana **vitrectomy** is a form of retinal surgery in which the **vitreous gel** which fills the **posterior segment** of the eye is removed with an instrument called an **ocutome**. Three small holes (ports) are made into the eye through the pars plana through which surgical instruments, a light source and a fluid irrigation line can be inserted. This **surgery** is used for **complex** retinal detachments, (see 16.16), advanced diabetic eye disease, macular holes (see 11.17) and for retrieving fragments of lens nucleus in complicated phaco cataract surgery (see 16.6).

16.18 Oculoplastic Surgery – Ectropion Repair

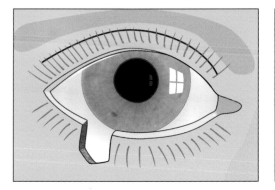

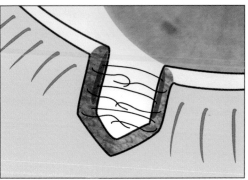

A piece of lid is excised to reduce the lid laxity and turn the lid in

The edges of the cut lid are sutured together carefully

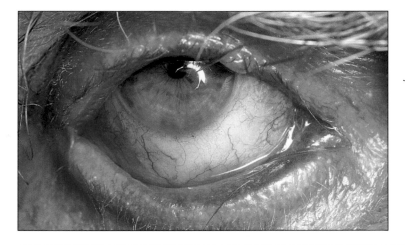

Ectropion – the lower lid edge is turned away from the eye

One of the main factors responsible for lower lid ectropion (see 6.4) is horizontal laxity of the lid. Most of the surgical approaches to ectropion correction involve a full thickness horizontal shortening of the lid (usually under local anaesthesia). Skin sutures are removed at about one week post-operation, but lid margin sutures need to be left in place for a further week to prevent notching of the margin at the repair site.

16.19 Oculoplastic Surgery – Entropion Repair

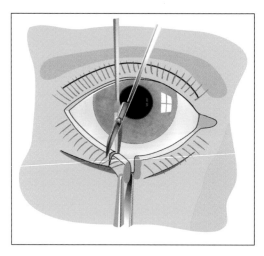

The lid is incised horizontally and section of lid is excised

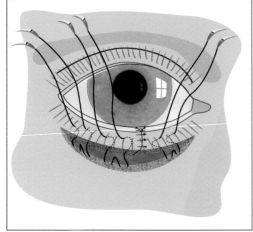

The lid is sutured carefully to shorten and rotate it away from the eye

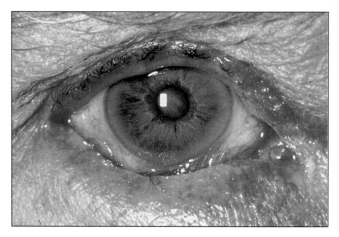

Entropion – the lower lid is rotated towards the eye, abrading it

Lower lid entropion repair often involves correcting both excess horizontal lid laxity and reduced effectiveness of the lower lid retractor complex. Full thickness **horizontal shortening** of the lid can be combined with **plication of the lid retractors** through a transverse skin incision.

16.20 Oculoplastic Surgery – Ptosis Repair

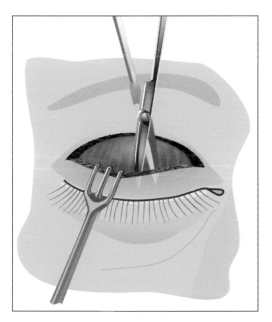

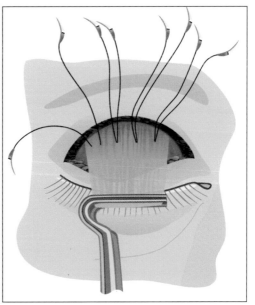

The upper eyelid is incised to expose the muscle which elevates the lid (levator palpebrae superioris)

The levator muscle is isolated and resutured to lift the lid

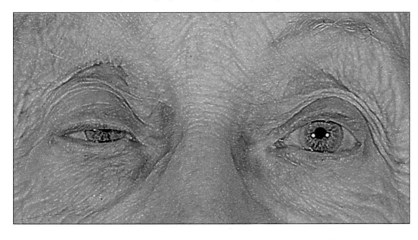

Ptosis – the right upper eyelid droops and covers the visual axis in this patient

Most senile ptosis is due to **dehiscence** of the levator palpebrae superioris aponeurosis (see 6.5). The aponeurosis is identified, repaired and reattached to the tarsal plate of the upper lid via a **skin crease incision**. Surgery is usually performed under **local anaesthesia**, so that the upper lid can be set at the correct height. Care must be taken in the early post-operative period to avoid **corneal exposure** from incomplete lid closure.

16.21 Incision and Curettage of Meibomian Cyst

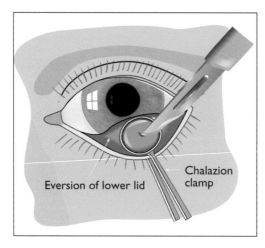

The lid is everted and a vertical linear incision is made in the cyst

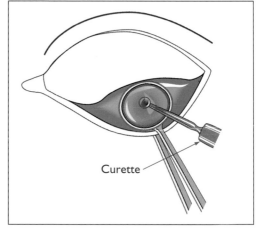

The contents of the cyst are curetted out

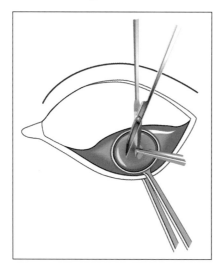

Granulation tissue formed from chronic inflammation may be excised

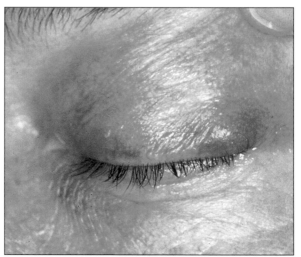

Chalazion – the external appearance is of a red inflamed lump in the lid

Incision and curettage (I+C) of Meibomian cysts is a commonly performed procedure for patients who have not responded to simple measures (see 6.9). After injection of local anaesthetic into the lid, the lid is everted with a special clamp and a linear incision is made through the tarsal conjunctiva into the cyst. The contents of the cyst are then curetted. The procedure is carried out under general anaesthesia in children.

16.22 Dacryocystorhinostomy

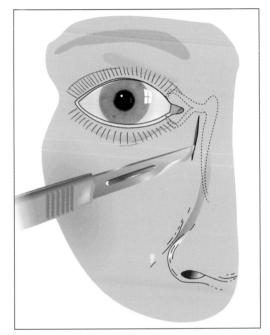

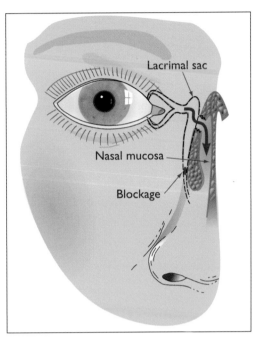

A skin incision is made to expose the lacrimal sac (dotted lines)

The lacrimal sac is anastomosed to the nasal mucosa

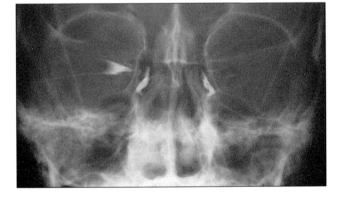

Dacryocystogram – X-ray with the lacrimal drainage system highlighted in white

The most common indication for a dacryocystorhinostomy (DCR) is **epiphora** with **blockage of** the nasolacrimal duct. The aim of the operation is to **bypass** the obstruction by anastomosing the lacrimal sac mucosa to the nasal mucosa. It is necessary to remove the bone separating the sac from the nose in order to do this. If there is a high chance of post-operative scarring, the newly created anastomosis can be intubated with **silicone tubes**, which stay in situ for at least 6 weeks. Recent advances in lacrimal surgery include using an endonasal approach with laser, although DCR remains the operation with the highest success rate at present.

16.23 Repair of Penetrating Eye Injury

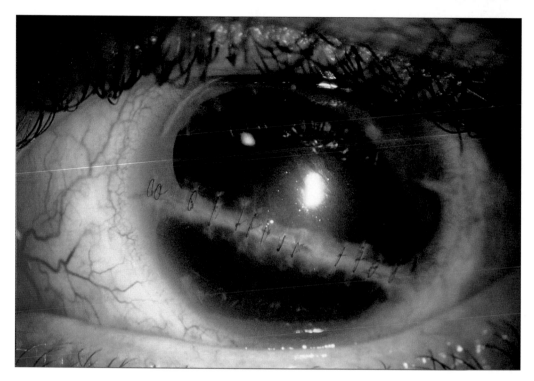

A laceration across the centre of the cornea has been repaired leaving a scar

With modern **microsurgical** techniques it is usually possible to restore the integrity of the globe and preserve useful vision in **even the most severe injuries** (see 7.5). After the primary repair, the eye is assessed carefully to determine the degree of damage, and the risk of **sympathetic ophthalmitis** developing in the other eye. Sympathetic ophthalmitis is an **autoimmune** disease associated with severe uveal trauma, in which a severe destructive reaction is mounted against the remaining good eye. **Early enucleation** (see 16.25) of a badly damaged eye largely eliminates this risk.

16.24 Semiconductor Diode Laser Ablation of the Ciliary Body

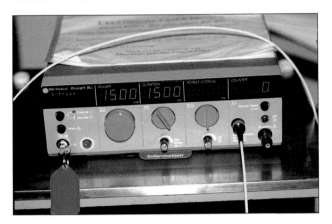

The diode laser is small and portable

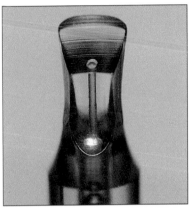

The laser probe is shaped to the eye with a fibreoptic cable for the laser light

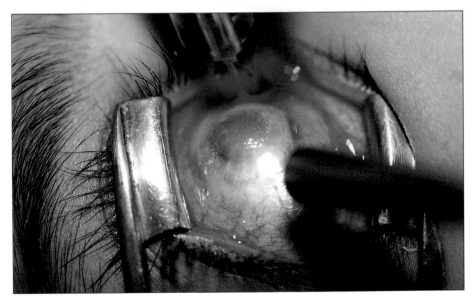

The ciliary body is identified by transillumination and then lasered

The management of persistently raised intraocular pressure in patients with **refractory glaucoma** has been aided by the development of **semiconductor diode laser cycloablation**. Aqueous production is decreased by the trans-scleral application of laser burns to the **ciliary body**. The treatment can be performed under either local or general anaesthesia as a **day-case**. The main advantage of the diode laser is the low incidence of complications. Treatment may be repeated several times.

16.25 Enucleation – Socket

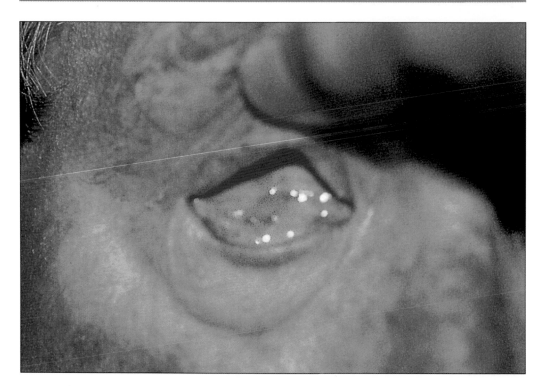

Post enucleation – socket without prosthesis

Surgical removal of an eye is a **major** procedure, and patients often experience feelings of **loss**, **depression** and uncertainty about the final **cosmetic** appearance. Enucleation is usually performed for intraocular malignancy, severe penetrating eye injuries (where there is a risk of sympathetic ophthalmitis) and for chronic ocular pain in eyes which are blind from a wide range of diseases. At the time of surgery a spherical **orbital implant** is inserted into the orbit, in order to replace the lost volume.

16.26 Enucleation – Prostheses

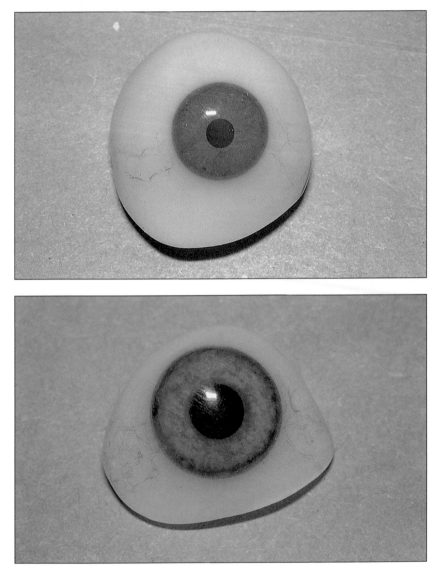

Range of prosthetic eye shells

It is important that one obtains a good fit for the cosmetic ocular prosthesis. Impression **moulding** of the remaining conjunctival sac after enucleation enables the technical team to fashion a prosthesis which is comfortable and symmetrical with the other eye. Prostheses can be matched for eye colour, pupil size and surface vascularity.

16.27 Enucleation – Fitted Prosthesis

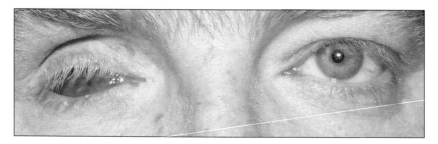

Enucleated socket

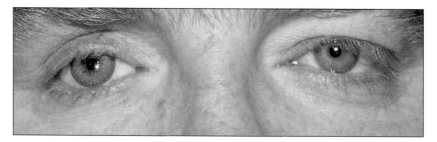

Prosthetic shell in situ

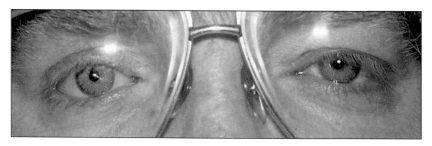

Spectacle correction enhances cosmetic appearance

When the conjunctival surface of the socket has healed a **cosmetic prosthetic shell** is fitted into the remaining conjunctival sac. The **orbital implant** placed into the orbit at the time of enucleation is designed to give the final prosthesis a reasonable degree of **movement**. After a prosthesis has been fitted, it is sometimes necessary to correct lower lid laxity or upper lid ptosis surgically in order to get the best fit and cosmesis.

16.28 Cosmetic Prosthetic Shell

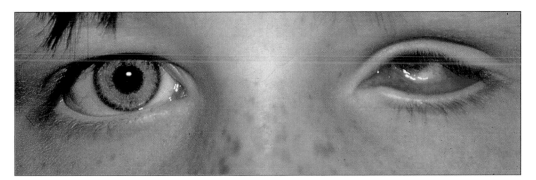

Microphthalmic left eye

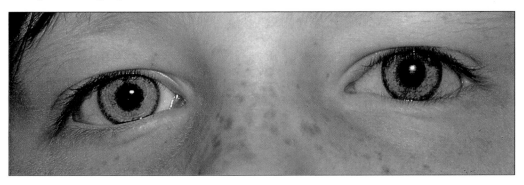

Cosmetic prosthetic shell in situ on top of microphthalmic left eye

The image above shows how a cosmetic prosthetic shell can be fitted over the **surface** of a blind (microphthalmic) eye producing excellent cosmesis. In order to achieve the best fit for the shell it may be necessary to correct any associated **lid malposition** (e.g entropion or ptosis).

Common Abbreviations

The following abbreviations are commonly used by ophthalmic specialists and are actively used in this book:

A-P	Antero-posterior	IOP	Intraocular pressure
AACG	Acute angle-closure glaucoma	JCA	Juvenile chronic arthritis
AAU	Acute anterior uveitis	KP	Keratic precipitate
AIDS	Acquired immunodeficiency syndrome	LA	Local anaesthetic
		LASIK	Laser in-situ keratomileusis
AION	Anterior ischaemic optic neuropathy	LGN	Lateral geniculate nucleus
		MMC	Mitomycin C
ARMD	Age-related macular degeneration	NPDR	Non-proliferative diabetic retinopathy
C/D	Vertical cup: disc ratio		
CF	Count fingers	NTG	Normal tension glaucoma
CFB	Corneal foreign body	Oc	Ointment
CMV	Cytomegalovirus	OM	Operating microscope
CNIII	Third cranial nerve	PCT	Prism cover test
CRAO	Central retinal artery occlusion	PDR	Proliferative diabetic retinopathy
CRVO	Central retinal venous occlusion	PI	Peripheral iridotomy
D	Dioptre	PL	Perception of light
DCG	Dacryocystography	POAG	Primary open angle glaucoma
DCR	Dacryocystorhinostomy	PRK	Photo-refractive keratectomy
DS	Divergent strabismus	PRP	Pan-retinal photocoagulation
ECCE	Extracapsular cataract extraction	PSCLO	Posterior subcapsular lens opacity
EOG	Electro-oculography	PVD	Posterior vitreous detachment
ERG	Electroretinography	RAPD	Relative afferent pupil defect
5-FU	5-Fluorouracil	ROP	Retinopathy of prematurity
FFA	Fundus fluorescein angiography	RP	Retinitis pigmentosa
G.	Guttae (eye drops)	SCC	Squamous cell carcinoma
HM	Hand movements	TED	Thyroid eye disease
HZO	Herpes zoster ophthalmicus	VEP	Visual-evoked potential
I+C	Incision and curettage	VER	Visual-evoked response
ICCE	Intracapsular cataract extraction	YAG	Yttrium-Aluminium-Garnet
IOL	Intraocular lens		

Differential Diagnosis of the Red Eye: 'The Top 50'

Orbit

Thyroid eye disease

Carotid-cavernous fistula

Arterio-venous malformation

Non-specific orbital inflammatory disease ('pseudotumour')

Lymphoproliferative diseases

Cavernous sinus thrombosis

Superior vena caval obstruction

Eyelids

Entropion

Ectropion

Trichiasis

Distichiasis

Chronic blepharo-conjunctivitis

Floppy eyelid syndrome

Eyelid imbrication syndrome

Canaliculitis

Lacrimal sac abscess

Molluscum contagiosum

Basal cell carcinoma

Sebaceous (Meibomian) gland carcinoma

Conjunctiva

Infective conjunctivitis (viral, bacterial, chlamydial)

Subtarsal foreign body

Subtarsal concretions

Subconjunctival haemorrhage

Dry eye syndrome

Cicatricial ocular pemphigoid

Trachoma

Rosacea

Stevens-Johnson syndrome

Conjunctiva (continued)

Allergic disease (Allergic conjunctivitis, Atopic keratoconjunctivitis)

Drug (e.g. preservative toxicity/ hypersensitivity)

Pterygium

Phlyctenular conjunctivitis

Pingecula

Superior limbic keratoconjunctivitis

Parinaud's oculoglandular conjunctivitis

Ocular surface squamous neoplasia

Cornea

Loose corneal suture

Herpetic keratitis (Epithelial, Stromal and Metaherpetic disease)

Zoster keratoconjunctivitis

Exposure keratopathy (Lagophthalmos in CNVII palsy)

Neurotrophic keratopathy

Bullous keratopathy

Contact lens-related keratopathy

Marginal keratitis

Peripheral ulcerative keratitis

Corneal abscess

Sclera

Episcleritis

Scleritis

Anterior Chamber

Uveitis (Anterior, Posterior, Panuveitis)

Acute angle-closure glaucoma

Neovascular glaucoma

Endophthalmitis (Post-operative, Endogneous)

acanthamoeba 65
accommodation 34, 35
acquired immunodeficiency
    syndrome (AIDS) 86
acrylic-based materials 146
acute corneal graft rejection 153
adenoviral keratoconjunctivitis 56
age-related maculopathy – drusen 103
alcohol abuse 13
alkaline agents 60
amblyopia 115, 118, 120, 123, 127, 128
amblyopia, occlusion therapy 118
Amsler chart 105, 106, 109
aneurysms 97, 132, 135, 136
angiogenic growth factors 80
anisocoria 139
ankylosing spondylitis 84, 85
antimetabolite, 5-Fluorouracil 150
antimetabolite, Mitomycin C 150
aphakia 92
applanation tonometry 23
arterial occlusion 80, 96
arterio-venous nipping 102
arthritis, rheumatoid 69, 71
arthritis, juvenile chronic 81
artificial tears 54
astigmatism 36, 148, 152
atrial fibrillation 96
autoantibodies 141
automated visual field 78
automated visual field testing 29
band keratopathy 81
Behçet's disease 84, 85
bifocal 35
binocular function 120
bleeding diathesis 72
blepharitis 44, 45, 64
blind registration 33, 99
blood pressure 72
blood-ocular barrier 32
blow-out fracture of the orbit 51
Bruch's membrane 103
buphthalmos 126
capsular bag 146, 148, 149
carcinoma, basal cell 37, 38
carcinoma, squamous cell 38
cataract 27, 36, 81, 87-89, 92, 107,
    123, 144, 146-9, 160
cataract, congenital 123
cataract surgery 144, 146-9, 160
central retinal artery occlusion 96
central retinal venous occlusion 80, 95,
    100, 101, 130
cerebrovascular events 18, 133, 140
chemical eye injury 60
cherry red spot 96

chiasm, chiasmal compression 18, 132
chiasm, optic nerve
    and chiasmal gliomas 132
chiasm, retro-chiasmal lesions 133
chlamydia trachomatis 121
choroidal folds 108
choroidal melanoma 111
choroidal metastatic deposit 112
choroidal naevus 113
cicatricial 39, 40, 42, 54, 70, 124
cicatricial disease 54
ciliary body 16, 167
cold sore 62
coloboma 27, 127
commotio retinae 110
cones 17
confrontation test (visual fields) 132
congenital nasolacrimal obstruction
    121, 126
conjunctiva 15, 40, 54, 55, 66, 67, 70,
    72, 150, 151
conjunctivitis 48, 55, 56, 66, 70, 121
conjunctivitis, adenoviral 56
conjunctivitis, allergic –
    giant papillae 66
conjunctivitis, bacterial 55
conjunctivitis, cicatricial –
    pemphigoid 42, 54, 70
conjunctivitis, infective 55
contact lens-related infection 65
cornea 13, 15-16, 23, 30, 36, 39, 40, 42,
    50, 56, 58, 62-5, 67, 70, 73, 80, 82, 84,
    121, 126, 137, 152-7
corneal abscess 65, 84
corneal dystrophies 152
corneal exposure 40, 50, 137, 163
corneal foreign body 58
corneal oedema 80
corneal scarring 42, 62, 70
corneal transplantation – penetrating
    keratoplasty 152, 153
corneal ulcer 42, 63-4
corneal ulcer, geographical 63
cortical lens opacity 89
cosmetic prosthetic shell 169-71
cotton wool spots 97, 102
cranial nerve palsy, fourth 135
cranial nerve palsy, seventh –
    lagophthalmos 40, 137
cranial nerve palsy, sixth 136
cranial nerve palsy, third 41, 134, 139
craniopharyngioma 132
cryotherapy 125, 159
cystoid macular oedema 107
cytomegalovirus 86
dacryocystitis 52
dacryocystography 53

dacryocystorhinostomy 52, 165
demyelination 31, 129, 136, 140
dendritic ulcer – herpes simplex
    keratitis 62-3
dermatitis, allergic 43
dermatitis, atopic 44
diabetes mellitus 85, 95, 97-101, 136
diathesis, bleeding 72
diplopia 51, 135-6, 141
distortion 89, 105-6
drainage angle 74, 80, 114
drug toxicity 129
drusen 103, 105, 113
drusen, hard 103
drusen, soft 103
dry eye syndrome 54, 70
ectopia lentis 91
ectropion 40, 137, 161
electro-oculography 31
electrodiagnostic tests 31, 107
electrolysis 42
electroretinography 31
emboli 96
embryology 13-14
endophthalmitis 84, 151
endophthalmitis, metastatic 84
endophthalmitis, post-operative 84
enophthalmos 51
entropion 39, 162, 171
enucleation 111, 166, 168-170
enucleation – prosthesis 169, 170
enucleation – socket 168
epilation 42
epiphora 40, 53, 137, 165
episcleritis 68
esotropia 115, 136
exotropia 116, 134
exudative diabetic maculopathy 98
flashes 93-4, 111-12
floaters 93-4, 101, 111-12
fluorescein 23, 32, 42, 62-3
foreign body, corneal 58
foreign body, intraocular 58, 138, 144
foreign body, subtarsal 57
fovea 17, 32, 96
Fuch's endothelial dystrophy 152
Fuch's heterochromic cyclitis 138
fundus fluorescein angiography 32
genetic counselling 107
giant cell arteritis 96, 131, 142
giant papillae 66
glaucoma 29, 33-4, 73-81, 83, 91, 95,
    114, 126 150, 167
glaucoma filtration surgery –
    trabeculectomy 150, 151
glaucoma, acute angle-closure 73, 75

Index

glaucoma, chronic angle-closure 75
glaucoma, infantile (buphthalmos) 126
glaucoma, neovascular 80, 95
glaucoma, normal (low) tension 79
glaucoma, open angle 33, 74, 79
glaucoma, primary open angle 74
glaucoma, pupil block 83
glaucoma, refractory 167
gonioscopy 74
gonococci 121
graft rejection 153
haemorrhage, peri-disc splinter 77, 131
haemorrhage, retinal 86, 95, 97, 102, 124
haemorrhage, subconjunctival 72
haemorrhage, vitreous 30, 101
haloes 73
head posture 135
hemianopia, bitemporal 132
hemianopia, homonymous 133
herpes simplex keratitis 62, 63
herpes zoster ophthalmicus 48, 138
heterochromia iridis 138, 140
Holmes-Adie syndrome 139
homocystinuria 91
Horner's syndrome 41, 138-140
hyaloid artery 13
hypercholesterolaemia 95
hyperlipidaemia 131
hypermetropia 34, 73, 75, 115
hypertension 95, 102, 130, 131
hypertension, malignant 102
hyperthyroidism 49
hyperviscosity 95, 131
hyphaema, traumatic 61
hypopyon 82, 84
hypothalamus 140
hypotropia 134
immunosuppressive therapy 70, 71
incision and curettage 164
infection, acanthamoebal keratitis 65
infection, AIDS 86
infection, conjunctivitis 55, 121
infection, contact lens-related 65
infection, corneal 65, 121, 157
infection, corneal abscess 65, 84
infection, cytomegalovirus 86
infection, dacryocystitis 52
infection, endophthalmitis
    (post-operative) 84, 151
infection, geographical corneal ulcer 63
infection, gonococci 121
infection, herpes zoster 48, 138
infection, herpes simplex 62, 63
infection, intrauterine 13, 123
infection, middle ear 136

infection, ophthalmia neonartorum
    121
infection, orbital cellulitis 46, 47
infection, paranasal sinus 47
infection, post-op bleb 151
infection, preseptal cellulitis 46
infection, retinal (retinitis) 86
infection, trachoma 42, 54
infection, tuberculosis 85
infection, viral 129
inflammatory bowel disease 85
inflammatory infiltrates 64
injury, penetrating 57-9, 92, 166, 168
intraocular foreign body 58, 138
intraocular lens 92, 146, 148, 149
intraocular pressure 22-4, 61, 77, 79,
    80, 150, 167
intraocular pressure phasing 79
iris 15, 16, 75
iris melanoma 114, 138
iris prolapse 59, 147
iris, lesion 114
iris, peripheral 75
iris, post-operative prolapse 147
irrigation 60, 160
ischaemic optic neuropathy 130, 131
ischaemic retina 80, 96, 100, 125
jaw claudication 142
juvenile chronic arthritis 81
keratic precipitates – sarcoidosis 82
keratitis 48, 62, 64-5
keratitis, adenoviral 56
keratitis, herpes simplex 62-3
keratitis, marginal 64
keratoconus 36, 152
keratoplasty, penetrating 152, 153
keratosis, actinic 38
lacrimal system 14, 15, 52-4, 121, 126,
    165
lacrimal gland 54
lagophthalmos 40, 137
laser, argon laser macular grid 98
laser, lasik 154
laser, argon laser pan-retinal
    photocoagulation 100
laser, photo-refractive keratectomy 156
laser, YAG laser peripheral iridotomy 75
laser, YAG laser posterior capsulotomy
    149
laser in-situ keratomileusis (lasik) 154
lateral geniculate nucleus 18
lazy eye 118
lens, 20 Dioptre 26
lens, 78 Dioptre 22
lens, cortical opacity 89
lens, crystalline 34-5, 87, 91

lens, cylindrical 36
lens, embryology 14
lens, intraocular 30, 92, 146, 148-9
lens, nuclear sclerosis 88
lens, posterior subcapsular opacity 90
leukocoria 27, 122, 123
levator palpebrae superioris muscle
    41, 128, 163
lid hygiene 44
lid lag 49
lid retraction 49
lipid exudate 97-8, 102
local anaesthesia 26, 145, 163
low birth weight 124
low visual aids 104
macula 17, 93, 98, 103-7, 109, 133, 160
macular disease 33, 106
macular hole 109, 160
maculopathy 97
maculopathy, age related – drusen 103
maculopathy, exudative diabetic 98, 103
maculopathy, exudative disciform 105
malingering 31
Marfan's syndrome 91
Meibomian cyst 45, 164
Meibomian glands 44, 45
melanoma, choroidal 111
metamorphopsia 104-6
metastasis 37-8, 112
microkeratome 154
microaneurysms 97
microphthalmos 127
microscope, operating 143
migraine 79
miosis 140
myasthenia gravis 41, 141
myasthenic crisis 141
myopia 33, 36, 88, 93, 156
nasal steps 78
nasolacrimal, obstruction 52, 55, 121,
    126, 165
nasolacrimal, dacryocystitis 52
nasolacrimal, dacryocystography 53
nasolacrimal, dacryocystorhinostomy
    165
nasolacrimal, duct 52-3, 121, 126, 165
night vision 107
non-exudative age-related macular
    degeneration 104
nuclear sclerosis 88
obstructive hydrocephalus 132
occipital cortex 18, 133
occlusion therapy, amblyopia 118
ocular hypotony 108
ocular ultrasonography 30, 87, 94
ophthalmia neonatorum 121

ophthalmoscopy, direct 25, 27
ophthalmoscopy, indirect 26
optic atrophy 129
optic chiasm 18, 132
optic disc 25, 76-7, 129-31
optic disc, atrophy 77, 107, 129
optic disc, glaucomatous cupping 77, 129
optic disc, papilloedema 130
optic disc, swollen 102, 130, 131
optic nerve and chiasmal gliomas 132
optic nerve head 16, 17, 30, 32, 77, 79, 129, 130, 131
optic nerve head, cupping of the 77
optic nerve, compression of the 18, 50
optic neuritis 130
optic neuropathy, ischaemic 130-1, 142
optic radiations 18
optic tract 18
optic vesicles 14
orbital cellulitis 46, 47
orbital implant 168, 170
orbital septum 46-7
orbital vascular anomaly 72
orthoptists 120
pan-retinal laser photocoagulation 100
papilloedema 130
paranasal sinuses 47
pemphigoid 42, 54, 70
penetrating eye injury 57-9, 92, 166, 168
peribulbar injection 145
peripheral iridotomy 75
phacoemulsification 144, 146, 148
phasing (of intraocular pressure) 79
photo-refractive keratectomy 156
photophobia 56, 64-5
pin-hole 19
pituitary tumours 132
pneumotonometry 24
Polymethylmethacrylate (PMMA) 146
post-herpetic neuralgia 48
posterior subcapsular lens opacity 90
posterior synechiae 83
posterior vitreous detachment 93-4, 101
preauricular lymphadenopathy 56
prematurity 124-5
presbyopia 35
preseptal cellulitis 46
preservative 43
prism cover test 119
proptosis 47, 49, 50
psoriasis 85
pterygium 67

ptosis 41, 128, 134, 140-1, 163, 170-1
ptosis, congenital dystrophic 128
pupil-block 75, 83
quadrantanopia, homonymous 133
radial keratotomy 157
Raynaud's phenomenon 79
red reflex 25, 27, 90, 122
refractive surgery, lasik (laser in-situ keratomileusis) 154
refractive surgery, photo-refractive keratectomy 156
refractive surgery, radial keratotomy 156
relative afferent pupil defect 87, 95
retina, embryology 14
retinal detachment 33, 91, 93, 94, 124, 149, 159, 160
retinal ganglion cells 18
retinal haemorrhage 86, 95
retinal tear 93, 94, 110
retinitis pigmentosa 107
retinitis, infective 86
retinoblastoma 27, 122
retinopathy of prematurity 124-5
retinopathy, hypertensive 102
retinopathy, non-proliferative diabetic 97
retinopathy, proliferative diabetic 80, 99-101
retinopathy, sickle cell 101
rheumatoid arthritis 69, 71
rosacea 42, 44
rubeosis iridis 80
sarcoidosis 54, 82, 84-5
Schirmer's test 54
sclera 15, 16, 71, 159
scleral explant 159
scleritis 69, 71, 108
scleromalacia perforans 71
scotomas, arcuate 78
scotomas, paracentral 78
secondary re-bleed 61
semiconductor diode laser cycloablation 167
siderosis 138
silicone 146, 159, 165
silicone tube intubation 165
slit-lamp 22-3, 82
Snellen Chart 19
stereopsis 120
strabismus 115-18, 120, 158
strabismus surgery 158
strabismus, convergent 115
strabismus, divergent 116
strabismus, vertical 117
subconjunctival haemorrhage 72

subtarsal foreign body 57
superficial temporal artery 142
suppression 120
suture adjustment 152
suture, microsurgical 144, 147, 153, 161-2
suture, 10/0 nylon monofilament 144
symblepharon 70
sympathetic innervation 140
sympathetic ophthalmitis 166, 168
synoptophore 120
syphilis 85
temporal artery biopsy 142
test, automated visual field 29
test, prism cover 119
test, Schirmer's 54
thyroid eye disease 49, 50, 108, 117, 119
tonometry, applanation 23
tonometry, pneumo 24
toxocara 122
trabecular meshwork, embryology 14
trabeculectomy 150-1
trachoma 42, 54
trauma, blow-out orbital fracture 51
trauma, commotio retinae 110
trauma, hyphaema 61
trauma, penetrating eye injury 59
trichiasis 42
tuberculosis 85
tumour, intraocular 80, 122
tumour, nerve 130, 134
tumour, orbital 108, 117
tumour, pigmented 114
tumour, pituitary 132
tumour, primary 112
ultrasonography 30, 87, 94
uveitis 48, 81-6
vasospastic diseases 79
vertical cup:disc ratio 76
visual (occipital) cortex 18, 133
visual acuity 19, 111, 130
visual field 18, 28, 29, 78, 93, 107, 111, 112, 132-3
visual pathway 18, 129, 133
visual-evoked potential 31
vitrectomy 109, 160
vitreous gel 16, 30, 94, 160
vitreous haemorrhage 27, 30, 101
vitreous, posterior detachment 93, 94, 101
wound dehiscence 147
YAG laser 75
YAG laser capsulotomy 149